Books by E-O-L Publishing Corporation

Dying with Joy and Sorrow
By Judy Voss and Linda Neider

More Joy Than Sorrow
By Judy Voss

Compassion & Joy
By Judy Voss

Compassion

& Joy

at the end-of-life

Compiled by Judy Voss

Cover design by Nikki Griffin
Rose bouquet by Don Welty

Printed in the United States of America for
E-O-L Publishing Corporation, a nonprofit organization,
PO Box 1341, New Smyrna Beach, FL 32170.
Proceeds from the sale of this book provide
continuing education for hospice end-of-life care.

Library of Congress Cataloging-in-Publication Data
Voss, Judy.
Compassion & Joy at the end-of-life
ISBN 978-0-9753705-1-3

This book is not intended to be a substitute
for professional medical or legal advice.

Com·pas·sion: *a feeling of deep sympathy for one who is suffering or stricken by misfortune, accompanied by a strong desire to relieve it*

Joy: *an especially ecstatic or exultant happiness for someone or something greatly valued or appreciated*

Contents

Chapter 3 End-of-Life Decisions *77*

Chapter 4 Just Past the Final Hour *89*

Pictures:

Foreword

    Within your hands is a compilation of true stories told by the dying, their family members, hospice staff, volunteers, and a variety of other caregivers. I can assure you that some stories will leave you with a feeling of great awe and some with thought provoking doubt. Either way, you will acquire a much greater awareness and understanding of what living while dying is really all about.

    If you have ever wondered what dying is like and how to care for someone who is approaching death, with or without hospice, then this book is for you. Those who anticipate a death or are in the midst of mourning will find solace in what others have already experienced, what helped them cope with grief, and what their thoughts are regarding an afterlife. Within these pages you will also learn about the funeral industry, what end-of-life decisions should be made, and find valuable resources that can assist you through the process of death, dying and bereavement.

    To honor those we have lovingly cared for and attended to in death, **Compassion and Joy** *embraces the outstanding beauty of the white rose as a symbol of remembrance of those who have passed before us. When the white rose rests amidst the red roses we are joyously reminded that even in death we are still together.*

Judy Voss

Dedication:

This book is dedicated to those who have shown great compassion for the dying and found joy in caring for those so loved. Through the sharing of their stories, others will be encouraged and not fear doing what some have so graciously and selflessly already done.

1 Prelude to Death & Dying

After kicking off my shoes, I crawled up on the king size bed where Jake lay on his left side. Countless times I have done the same maneuver but somehow this time felt a little different, more serene. The bedroom was filled with a sense of peace as if a burden had been lifted from within and yet saddled with an intense grief.

Glancing over Jake's right shoulder while kneeling behind him, I noticed precious family photos on the wicker stand an arm's length away and just steps from that sat a bedside commode. His very attentive and loving wife Elisabeth positioned herself at the edge of their bed she and Jake had just shared for the last time. Tears were cascading down her cheeks from heartache and sorrow only a widow could understand as she waited for me to determine if he had really and truly died.

When married sixty-seven years ago in a little hamlet town in New England, Jake and Elisabeth would have never imagined their final days and hours together on earth would end like this. They never expected one would be providing such intimate care for the other and somehow find joy in doing it and compassion in sharing it. But with a team of hospice staff and volunteers assisting Jake and Elisabeth, he was able to die at home where he wanted, the way he wanted, and with whom he wanted.

To the skeptic, I say, "You are right! Death doesn't always look like this." None of us will die the same way Jake did but most of us can die in peace and surrender as he did with loving arms wrapped around him. Together let us go on a journey that Jake and Elisabeth have already traveled, along with many others, so we will be more familiar with what it is like to be a caregiver of the dying, whether it is caring for your loved one, a patient in a health care facility, your neighbor, your pet, or even yourself, and what you may expect as death approaches. Most of us have purposely avoided this topic so let us loosen our tongues, our hearts, and our souls and confront death because avoiding it is not an option for any of us.

Language of Death

Because death and dying has long been a taboo subject, consequently it has been laden with its own language of avoidance through the use of euphemisms. Euphemisms or slang terms have been associated with death and dying as long as words have been recorded. Saying one is *passed away* is a kinder and more gentle way to say one has died, especially when the news is so fresh. We use gentler words because they are less threatening and provide some distancing of death before the full impact can be grasped or comprehended. Especially with children, words should be chosen carefully so as not to convey one who has died as being *asleep* or *lost* which would add more confusion and distress to the child when the reality of the permanence of their loved one's death is realized.

What somewhat disturbs me is the acceptance and highly anticipated décor of Halloween being laden with characters depicting gruesome deaths, ghoulish skeletons, and horrific sound effects, as if that is the true depiction of death and dying. A frightening statistic that is also disturbing is that before children complete elementary school it is estimated that each views over 8,000 murders and 10,000 acts of violence on television and in movies. Also viewed are countless cartoon characters who experience violent acts that would undoubtedly cause death, yet each recovers without ill effects.

So why is a natural, peaceful and anticipated death not honestly and openly discussed until absolutely necessary and why is the deathbed scene tucked behind closed doors? Perhaps we need an attitude adjustment.

Adjusting our Attitude

The avoidance of discussing death and dying may be related to our fears of the unknown. The uncertainties can be many such as the anticipation of suffering or pain, concerns over one's dignity being maintained, wondering if death will come during sleep or in wakefulness, will death occur at home, will death come when we are alone, will we be in a comatose or vegetative state, and/or will concerns of life after death or any unfinished business impede the hope of having a peaceful death. Unrealistically, perhaps we hold onto the thought that we may be the first immortal one and so death is not of any concern, which is certainly classified as *death denying*. If we don't talk about it then it won't happen, right? Wrong.

Undoubtedly it will be necessary for you at least once in your lifetime to be a caregiver and attend to the dying whose needs must be placed before your own. I guarantee you that providing care for the dying will change you... for the better. Yet even the thought of being a caregiver of the dying can cause anxiety, perhaps a severe *death anxiety*. Yet the concerns I mentioned can be anticipated and probably easily surmounted by learning as much as we can before our care giving is needed. If one's death is anticipated by a physician to occur within a six month time period then a hospice team can provide invaluable assistance to the dying and their families or friends who are caregivers. (You will learn more about hospice care in Chapter Two.)

Sally Fields recently starred in an excellent movie titled *Two Weeks* that portrays how her adult children adapt to her approaching death and the care they and hospice provide. Another great movie about death and dying is *The Bucket List,* featuring Morgan Freeman and Jack Nicholson, a story of two dissimilar friends who live their lives to the fullest in their last days together. I highly recommend you view both..

Saying Good-bye

There are many compassionate caregivers on this earth. One very astute caregiver is Melissa Malcolm. She is a Certified Nursing Assistant/CNA who cares for hospice patients in nursing facilities. Thankfully Melissa recognized her patient's death anxiety and what he really needed before his death. Then she fulfilled his wish through a simple act of kindness. Here is Melissa's story:

I had a patient a year ago who came on the hospice program and he was a little demanding and somewhat hard to get along with. I would see this gentleman two to three times a week and it seemed like each time I would visit the harder it would be to get along with him. This gentleman had the nursing home staff beside themselves, making it hard for them to even want to check on him and just dreading to hear what he may say. I would often think what on earth could I do for this man to make his last days happy. Then it dawned on me.

I remembered I went to a CNA meeting one time and the Coordinator Elsie spoke to the CNAs and gave us some advice, which I took. She told us that when a patient is hateful to people there is a reason why. Elsie said to try asking the patient if there is something bothering him or her and if there is anything I could do to help and usually they will open up. Well, I did just that.

One day I went into the patient's room and he was so nasty to me. I sat down by his bedside and said very softly and nicely, "What can I do to help you or make you happy?" He stared right at me and the tears started rolling. He told me he had a calling card and a telephone line hook up in his room. All he wanted was a telephone to call his sister in Alaska to tell her good-bye because he was ready to die.

I went to a nearby store and bought him a telephone, brought it back, and hooked it up. He was so happy he smiled at me, told me he was grateful, kissed my hand and said. "God bless you." The next evening my patient passed away.

As with Melissa's patient, sometimes death anxiety is hard to recognize because it may be disguised in an unlikely manner so it may take an unusual approach and an extra dose of compassion to overcome it. With all probability, the longer we live the more comfortable we should become in life and death simply by having more opportunities to experience both. Each individual's acceptance and approach to the dying, from cautiously standing in the hallway, to sitting at the bedside, to crawling up on the bed, will progress and regress according to our level of comfort, understanding and acceptance.

Lessons in Listening

Education is a very powerful tool so by listening well and reading countless resources available we can learn volumes that may be vital in meeting the needs of the dying. With your new knowledge you may recognize that a request for help to the bathroom because of extreme weakness may also be a cry for understanding as to why assistance is now needed. Sometimes just being present and sharing special moments in silence is enough. Kathy Sullivan explains it best:

What a guy! I met Stephen while working the evening shift as an Administrative Secretary in the Hospice Care Center. Stephen was a resident of Washington D.C. but, because of his terminal condition, he moved closer to his family in Florida and eventually lived at the Care Center. Stephen was a kind, soft-spoken, intelligent young man who studied and taught Shakespeare in Washington before he became ill.

Every evening, at about the same time, Stephen would slowly walk to the nurses' station with his cane in hand, stand in the doorway and ask me, "Is it time to lock the front door yet?" I was the person that locked the door every evening to ensure the Care Center staff knew what visitors desired entry after hours. This ritual continued every night until the time came that Stephen was too weak to take our memorable nightly walk.

I learned an unforgettable lesson during Stephen's stay at the Care Center that taking those leisurely walks to lock the front door each night was not about locking the front door at all.

When Children Talk

Our children can teach us immeasurable things if we heed their words. There are books full of stories told by children who have envisioned and predicted their death with pure certainty and a calm acceptance. One such book is *A Window To Heaven* by Diane M. Komp, M.D., who is a pediatric oncologist. Her little patients who were faced with dying voiced to her a great comfort in an understanding of a better life hereafter, a life they anticipated spending with Jesus. Dr. Komp heeded the words her children shared with her when they voiced the timeliness of their death, which helped her reclaim her own faith, and became a better listener and believer of little ones.

Truth Telling or Not

Whether we realize it or not, there are certain ways we tend to communicate, or not communicate, sad or happy news to others. Perhaps for a period of time we choose to keep secret an anticipated divorce, a probable job change, a move away from our parents, or a loss of income. We may prolong keeping these secrets for various reasons but generally it is to protect others from premature or potential sadness or grief.

There is much we can learn from those who are dying by the way they communicate to us. If we pay close attention to what they say, hear, or see we may discover they have a clear understanding of their approaching death. Some can predict the hour and day they will die with amazing accuracy. Many who are approaching death have an awareness of their final days and hours and may even sense or envision the presence of their deceased loved ones, angels, or other celestial presence. This understanding is known as *Near Death Awareness*.

Not everyone believes that death should be openly discussed as Sociologists Barney Glaser and Anselm Strauss have discovered. They address four styles of communication that are specific to death and dying, which they discuss in their book *Awareness of Dying*.

The first communication style is called *closed awareness* where others may know about one's approaching death but the one dying is purposely not informed. It may be believed that decisions regarding medical care should be decided on by the family so patient involvement and their awareness of their own death is not believed essential. Others may feel it is the will of God to let an illness progress so the information is not shared with the afflicted.

The second style of communication is known as *suspected awareness* where the ill person may sense their death approaching but it is still not openly discussed or verified by others. Perhaps loved ones of the dying feel it is best that the very ill not be burdened with sad news prematurely.

Next is *mutual pretense* where everyone including the dying is aware of one's approaching death but the subject is still avoided. Some feel that talking about death or beginning hospice care may cause death to transpire earlier or diminish any hope of remission. This style is similar to the adage of having an elephant in your living room yet everyone avoids talking about something so obvious. Dying is generally not a secret to the dying, even if others think it is. Just ask them and they will tell you that.

Finally, with *open awareness* an honest discussion of an approaching death between the dying, their loved ones, their caregivers and any others involved in end of life decisions is permissible and encouraged. This style allows the sharing of needs and concerns of the dying and of those who provide care, plus it provides time for closure and completion of life's details that may not have been addressed. In families with estranged loved ones, this extra time allows an opportunity to reunite and make amends. Another advantage of *open awareness* is the opportunity to complete Advance Directives, which are discussed in Chapter Three.

As a caregiver, it is imperative that one recognizes that certain cultures may have their own style of communication that may not allow open discussion of death and dying. It is with respect that caregivers must honor these requests of silence and deliver compassionate and nonjudgmental care to all.

Jake and Elisabeth, the couple referred to at the beginning of this chapter, used *open awareness* throughout his illness, as that is what they practiced throughout their marriage. Jake received hospice care for four months so many of his and his families' anxieties were addressed early on. Their open communication allowed their adult children time for visits and to assist in his care giving, plus it provided Jake a peace of mind in knowing that his wife would be well cared for after his death.

Our Life's Book

Our life is like a book. We all have our own autobiography tucked inside. Some books are of much greater length than others and some are sadly way too short. Most of us who live within the borders of more developed countries will have many chapters between our opening and closing ones. Contrary to what some may think, money cannot buy any of us extra chapters even if we try to bargain with God. We may get a few extra closing lines added to our book, with the help of some amazing medical interventions, but that's about the best we can expect and hope for.

However, if you believe in an afterlife than you know there is a sequel to your earthly book. Chapter Six will give you a peek into an anticipated afterlife.

There are many other books and articles that can help you in the writing of your own book of living and dying and prepare you to be better caregivers. These authors or researchers who have studied death and dying are called thanatologists. They have provided us with countless texts, life studies, and life experiences to better prepare us for dying and death, as well as for the grief work that is a critical part of recovery. Because my background is in nursing, I will briefly mention two thanatologists that I studied more closely. Others have been referenced for this book and are noted throughout the text and in the references in the back.

In 1959, Cicely Saunders first began writing about the needs of the dying. Her holistic approach in caring for the dying addressed not only her patients' physical needs but also their spiritual, psychosocial and familial needs. By far her legacy is the founding in 1967 of the world-renowned international hospice training facility called *St. Christopher's Hospice* near London, England, which I was so blessed to have been able to visit.

The author that my nursing career began with in 1971 was Elisabeth Kubler-Ross. She is best known for her tremendous compassion for those approaching death, plus her five stages of dying that she disclosed in her 1969 book titled On *Death and Dying*. She recognized that her dying patients were intermittently confronted and challenged by denial, anger, depression, bargaining and acceptance as their death approached.

The greatest of thanatologists are by far my patients. Each has made me more compassionate and understanding of what truly is needed as death approaches. They have taught me not to fear death but seek the joy that is plentiful even at the bedside of the dying. My patients have empowered me to share with you the best of what they have taught me, as well as stories shared by many others.

I encourage you to study and learn all you can from those who have traveled through life with the dying and with those who are grieving. There are countless resources available on the web or at your library, numerous death education courses available at many colleges and universities, and many associations and organizations that address the needs of the dying and those bereaved, many you will find in the back of the book.

It is now time to take the next brave step into Chapter Two and discover what dying is really like. My prayer is you will gain a greater appreciation for living by sharing in the lives of the dying and those who compassionately and joyously cared for them.

2 Caring for the Dying- With or Without Hospice

What do you think dying looks like, feels like, smells like, tastes like, and sounds like? What are the greatest concerns that those dying and their loving caregivers have? How does one know when death is close? We can learn so much from those who have experienced an approaching death of their own and by those who have cared for them. It is time to share in their most passionate end-of-life hours.

Lie in my bed

Imagine yourself dressed in a hospital gown, lying in a hospital bed covered with colorless sheets, side rails enclosed around you, barren walls glaring back at you, and fluorescent lights staring down upon you. There is a side table just out of your reach, heavily burdened with a bottle of generic lotion, an emesis basin, several mouth swabs, a plastic cup, a water pitcher and a meal tray with foul-smelling pureed foods begging to be touched. Attached to one side rail is your only connection to the outer walls, a bell to push with the hopes of a timely response before your bladder spills over or your pain returns. On the wall at the foot of your bed hangs a dry erase board with unfamiliar names to whom your care has been entrusted *yesterday*. Hanging precariously from the ceiling is a television that drones news that depresses the healthy and certainly the ill.

In the bed by the window lies a gentleman who is an arm's reach away. He has not spoken a word in the two days you have shared your whitewashed room and no family or friend has visited him. It is difficult to befriend someone under these circumstances with very few clues to rely on. With his oxygen machine hissing 24/7, any attempt at napping is near futile.

Outside the door you hear the alarming of machines begging for attention, frequent clanging noises from an assortment of delivery carts and stretchers, and call bells ringing and ringing and ringing.

Your most urgent thought and plea to your physician who has informed you that you may have four months to live is, "Can I please go home to die?" You have appreciated the care that you have received in the hospital but now home is where you want to be, where you want to die.

Less than twenty-four hours later, your wish has been granted and you are home under the care of hospice. So now what happens…

The Many Hands of Hospice

When many people hear the word hospice they think of death fast approaching, maybe even within just a few hours or a few days. In actuality, hospice care is available for those of all ages whose physician determines one's life expectancy is six months or less. However, dying is not so predictable and so patients may require hospice care for approximately a year or even more. A patient may stabilize while on hospice and the physician, together with the patient, caregivers, and hospice staff, may decide hospice care is not needed and so he/she will be discharged. However, hospice care can be resumed when needed in the future.

When I discuss hospice care with those not familiar, the vast majority of them have thought that hospice is mainly for patients who have cancer but that is not so. Approximately fifty percent of hospice patients have cancer and others have heart disease, kidney failure, Alzheimer's or Parkinson's Disease, AIDS, lung disease, liver disease, failure to thrive, Lou Gehrigs Disease, Multiple Sclerosis, etc. One of the main focuses of hospice is to improve one's quality of life by providing palliative care, which addresses the control of pain or other symptoms, for whatever the disease process may be.

As a hospice patient, you will be provided an interdisciplinary team of professionals who will address specific needs that you or your loving caregivers may have as you approach your death. Team members will visit you regularly and in emergency situations, addressing your physical, spiritual, emotional and psychosocial concerns and needs. Nurses, Social Workers, Chaplains, Home Health Aides and Certified Nursing Assistants, Volunteers, Complementary Therapists, Physical Therapists, Physicians, Bereavement Counselors, and countless support staff are available as part of hospice care. A whole new and positive outlook on truly living your final days has emerged with the expertise of a professionally trained and choreographed hospice team.

Despite the news of your approaching death, your terminal illness you were confronted with in the hospital looks, feels, smells, tastes, and sounds completely different in your beloved home. While lying in your own bed, covered with linens the shade of plums, you no longer are wearing a hospital gown but pajamas familiar and comfortable, surrounded by your very attentive family, as your cat stretches out at the foot of your bed. Your bedroom walls are graced with a soothing honey color, and photos of smiling and loving faces look down upon you. The person lying beside you is the one you have loved and cherished for many years, the one who knows your likes and dislikes, the one destined years ago to be your caregiver in sickness and in health and to forever love and to cherish.

If your physical needs require it and you so desire, hospice can provide home medical equipment that may provide more comfort and allow ease in providing physical care. The same kind of hospital bed and side table that are in hospitals can be supplied in the home. Other potentially needed medial equipment may include a commode, oxygen, nebulizer for breathing treatments, wheelchair, walker, or cane.

Another benefit to hospice patients is the medications their doctor orders that relate to their terminal illness can be provided through hospice, providing a significant financial savings. Each patient has their own doctor who orders the medications needed and follows the patient while receiving hospice care. A specialty trained hospice doctor may be available for consult and may be requested to provide care also.

Choosing a Care Giver

In my end-of-life class, the first question I ask of my attendees is *who do you want with you when you are dying?* Many of them had never given it a thought nor realized the significance in choosing. Do you realize how important it is for that certain someone (or two or three) to know they may be the chosen one to be at your bedside?

Family and close friends become a critical component for the dying, especially if they wish to die at home. I have seen adult sons and daughters tenderly care for their mothers and fathers. But I have also seen close friends and neighbors, grandchildren, stepchildren, church members, nieces and nephews, in-laws and perhaps, unknown to me, reformed outlaws providing care.

The chosen ones are sometimes those you would least expect. What care giving is really all about is who is at your bedside willingly, who has the privilege of being there, for that is truly what it is.

The Best in a Friend

I received an email several years ago that said God would send us carefully chosen friends depending on what we needed at the time. For example, if you are having a tough time with your teenager, He will send you a friend who also has a teenager and understands what troubles you are having and can provide you with support. If your car breaks down in the wee hours of the morning, it may be just minutes from a friend who has the ability to tow you home. Perhaps your mother has taken ill and you are concerned about a new medication she is taking so you call your friend who is a pharmacist. Bingo! You are a recipient of God's chosen friend!

You may not truly discover who your best friends, loved ones, or closest family members are until you are lying in your deathbed. They are the ones who compassionately provide intimate care when needed, be a sincere spokesperson when the dying is unable, and sit vigil as death approaches. These exceptional caregivers want to learn as much as they can about death and dying so they can provide the best of care to a loved one or patient. Those caring for you may become your voice when you cannot be understood and a trustworthy advocate to speak on your behalf, whether it is to a doctor, nurse, lawyer, family member, landlord, etc.

When it comes to the bedside of the dying, you can spot a best friend from the doorway or over the phone lines. She or he may be a neighbor, a classmate, a co-worker, a sister or brother, an aunt or mother, a spouse… someone who is willing to lovingly care for you at the end of your life. It touches me emotionally when I visit my hospice patients and there sits their best friend next to the bedside holding their hand, changing the linens on their bed or cleaning the commode, helping them figure out what to eat so they won't be sick and then try to fix it. These best friends may be performing manicures or helping with a shower, gently placing their best friend in a wheelchair and taking them for a stroll outside, or rubbing their achy back with soothing lotion. If times seem too tough to handle then your best friend may pray with you and ask for God's comfort and guidance in your care giving. These are the chosen ones that won't expect or want anything in return, except to be your friend.

The Missing Caregiver

The challenges and responsibilities of raising a family and tending to their needs are of utmost importance and no matter how much we wish we could temporarily walk away to care for someone else it just sometimes cannot be done. It is important to recognize and accept that these situations or personal responsibilities take priority. Certainly I would not expect someone with a child to forfeit his or her care for mine. Social Workers can be a great asset for families who need assistance and guidance in choosing in-home care or facility placement, if needed.

The Miraculous Little Seahorse

There are many homes away from home where those approaching death reside, short-term or long-term, and are able to receive hospice care. In hospitals, nursing homes, assisted living facilities, private residential homes or shelters, or hospice care centers are where hospice patients also reside. You may have a Hospice Care Center or Home in your neighborhood and not recognize it as such. It may look more like a five star hotel or resort. Once you step inside of a hospice house or care center, it may seem more like a loving home with overstuffed couches and chairs, a fireplace, piano, magazines and books, games, and a tray of cookies and sweets. A Chapel and/or Memorial Garden may be available, which provides a place for private prayer and reflection. Patient rooms are decorated in a home-like fashion but with all the necessities those approaching death may need. On the walls and on the dressers are momentoes and pictures from one's home, giving the feeling of belonging.

In any of these *homes*, you may be blessed to meet a compassionate and loving hospice volunteer, all of whom I hold in the highest regard. Hospice volunteer, Bobbie Hespelein, shares her touching story as she attended to her patient Randel Hamilton in a home away from home:

In Anchorage, Alaska, a heartbroken mother and father grieve for their firstborn, #1 son, Randy, who went home to the Lord May 1, 2007 at Hospice Care Center in Port Orange, Florida. Cancer claimed the life of this forty-eight-year-old gentle giant who was an aerial photographer in Alaska and Florida. He left behind a lovely wife Francey and three beautiful children.

It was humbling to be the hospice volunteer lending support to Randy, his wife Francey and family. I listened to his lovely mother, Fae, relive parts of Randy's childhood and their treasured time spent together through wonderful stories.

One afternoon Fae beckoned me to follow her outside Randy's room. Just outside she stopped and turned. Her eyes fell on the beautiful tile art plaque on the wall beside his door. Then, with palm outstretched, she began to trace over and over again with fingers, a pink seahorse titled "Reflections." The hues in the plaque were of great importance to her. Fae explained that pink represented courage and yellow represented cancer. There was a yellow cancer bracelet encircling her wrist.

Then Fae turned to me, focusing her eyes on mine, and said, "Bobbie, I hope I'm not going to shock you." She reached down, folded back her slacks, revealing her leg that had a small tattoo above her ankle- an exact replica of the little seahorse imprinted in colors of pink and yellow. Underneath it read #1.

I fought back the tears and told Fae that I thought her tattoo was a most beautiful gesture of love for her son. She went on to tell me that she and her daughters wore this same tattoo, imprinted while they were here in April to visit Randy at the Hospice Care Center. The deep inspiration conveyed from this small tile seahorse to Randy's mother was profound, personally meaningful and all encompassing. It symbolized Randy's life and his agonizing three-year battle with cancer, borne with great courage. It represented the room where Randy spent the last eight weeks of his prematurely aborted life, being cared for so gently by hospice nurses and staff.

Beautiful tile seahorse, you have bestowed upon Randy's mother an inspirational gift of rainbow colored memories, which will be with her always.

In memory of Randy and to honor his loving family and the hospice volunteer who compassionately cared for him, I have enclosed a picture of the seahorse plaque on page 70.

The Power of Pets

There is an open door policy with hospice care when it comes to their patients being visited by their beloved pets. Each has their own way of bringing comfort and joy through their unconditional love. They also provide snuggles we could all benefit from. Pets have a great sense as to when their loved one is approaching death, often displayed by their increased attentiveness or protectiveness of their master.

If a patient does not have a pet, hospice staff and volunteers will frequently bring his or her own to brighten a patient's day. That is what a hospice volunteer did with her Jack Russell Terrier dog on this very memorable day as told by Romane Casteel:

When the telephone call came to the hospice office, a concerned caregiver was worried about her patient, as she appeared not to respond to anyone or anything. She had one last idea that she thought just might work.

18

"Does any of your volunteers have a dog, a dog that is gentle?" the caregiver asked. "If so, would that person consider bringing the dog to the house to meet with my patient?"

The response was a "yes" knowing that a hospice volunteer had a Jack Russell Terrier dog named Jennie that might be able to help. So the dog's owner Mary was called and with her friend Elizabeth and her dog Jennie they set out on a mission they hoped would have a happy ending.

Mary explains what happened, "When we got to the home, we were ushered into a pleasant looking bedroom. The patient was lying comatose on the bed. Elizabeth and I looked at each other wondering if we were too late. There was no movement, no acknowledgment that someone had come into the room.

The caregiver said we could put Jennie on the bed. Cautiously I moved toward the bed and laid Jennie down. The little dog stood up and started moving around. Nothing happened. Then Jennie moved toward the patient's hand. She sniffed the hand and rubbed her nose in it. We thought we saw a finger move.

Suddenly, without warning, the patient sat straight up! It was a quick, strong movement much like you would have expected Lazarus to have made when he was raised from the dead. It all happened so fast- we were totally mesmerized!

The patient started talking haltingly to the dog. After she was convinced that she really had a four-legged friend on the bed with her, she whipped her legs around and while facing us began talking, not only to her caregiver but to Elizabeth and I as well.

It was a moment that we shall never forget, a wonderful experience to share with a friend. The caretaker was so thrilled that she is going to find a small dog to move in with her patient. Needless to say, this is one story that truly had a happy ending!"

On page 71 is a picture of this amazing and adorable Jack Russell Terrier dog that has brought joy to many.

Brown Cardinal

There are caregivers of all shapes and sizes, young and old, with and without feathers. Whoa! Wait a minute! What could I possibly mean by that? Well, author Rebecca Carpenter shares her inspirational story about a caregiver who we may not initially consider as such but I am sure you will change your mind. Rebecca tells it best:

With the sun barely up, I sat quietly in the dim light watching the lake. Subdued colors framed the dark water when I suddenly spotted a burst of bright color. My favorite birds perched at the edge of the feeder. The brilliant scarlet male cardinal then nestled in a bright green pine tree like a red bulb on a Christmas tree.

He was joined by his mate as they sat together, grabbed a bite to eat, and then quickly flew away. I had always thought that the females should be more colorful, but when I watched her spread her wings, I caught glimpses of red amidst the golden brown. She was not quite as plain as I had always believed. When they stood on the pine with wings slightly spread, their colors blended, and I realized how perfectly they complemented each other. God did not make a mistake in how they were colored. It was all part of His plan for the male to distract predators while the female was less noticeable and thus offered protection for the young. Each had a purpose as they worked together.

That same principle applies to people. It is easy to think that we should be the beautiful, talented, outgoing one who is the center of attention. However, each person who is in the limelight needs a supporting cast to assist and encourage them.

Our roles may change according to specific circumstances and periods of our lives. Wherever we have been placed, we need to do our job to the best of our ability to fulfill God's plan. We might be the teacher in front of the class or the custodian who cleans the room each day. We might be the preacher in the pulpit or the usher at the door of the church. We might be the doctor performing operations or the aide emptying bedpans. We might be the dad at a job supporting his family or the mother who is home raising the children. We might be leading a Christian crusade in a huge stadium or a missionary far from home sharing a Bible with a resident of a squatters' camp. The list could go on and on. As we journey through life, we must recognize our specific roles, perform our duties willingly as though working for Jesus, and be prepared for the next important assignment.

A Holy Coincidence

The majority of my hospice visits are completed during the weekend when my patients need symptom management, caregivers need support or education in how to best care for their loved one, or upon one's death. Typically every Sunday morning in Central Florida is sunny and this day was no different. The day began as usual but transpired rather quickly into what I call a *holy coincidence,* as a higher power than I had to be at the helm.

To begin any of my workdays as a hospice nurse, I first must connect the hospice laptop computer I carry with me to the main computer so I am assured of the most up to date information about my patients. On this one particular Sunday morning, I was not able to send or receive the information I needed via my laptop. Because I had patients waiting to be seen, it was decided that I would have to leave my laptop behind in the hospice office so the hospice office staff could troubleshoot it for me.

Upon obtaining my initial assignment of three patients and acquiring the medical supplies I anticipated needing, I headed to my van earlier than expected to begin my day. My initial patient needed a fasting blood sample drawn so I would go there first before she would eat her breakfast. However, just as I was preparing to leave the parking lot, the hospice triage nurse Diane phoned from the office I just left and said the patient called, wanted to eat breakfast now, and would not wait for my arrival. The patient chose to have the blood work completed the next day instead. So I was to continue on to my next patient.

My second patient, who had just been admitted to hospice the day prior, was twenty-five miles away so I arrived at his home approximately thirty minutes later. After assessing my patient, providing some personal care and education, and clarifying his medication needs with him and his caregivers, I proceeded to my third patient who was only a few miles down the road.

As I approached my next patient's home, the front yard was very welcoming with colorful flowers along the tidy stone walkway leading me to the front door. Just several feet inside lay my patient in a hospital bed. This gentle man greeted me with a cheery hello and immediately voiced his gratefulness for being home after so many days in the hospital. His wife reported he was doing much better than she had expected after his severe illness and was so relieved.

Just an hour prior to my arrival, my patient's wife reported he had combed his hair, washed his own face, and was thoroughly enjoying his time at home with his adored wife, his son, daughter-in-law and granddaughter who had just recently arrived from out of state, plus his very beloved little dog. After their dog yipped at me for several minutes, he recognized I wasn't a threat to his ailing master so he settled and accepted my presence. Together the family spoke of their life together, their love for the Lord, and how they missed attending their local church where many of their longtime friends were at this very hour. She expressed her thankfulness that their pastor visited the day prior and they expected church members to stop in and visit after the service was completed this morning.

The next twenty minutes I remember very clearly.

The main purpose of my visit was to redress a simple surgical wound for this gentle man. After assessing his vital signs and gathering my medical supplies, I began with his dressing change. I noticed the time we began was 11:00 a.m. just as their church service would have begun.

During the next ten minutes, his daughter-in-law, who is also a nurse, assisted me as I changed his dressing and then straightened his linens. As I was completing his care, this gentleman's breathing began to change. He developed a wet juicy sound in the back of his throat and could speak only a few words at a time due to his shortness of breath. He was very calm and had no fear or pain exhibited on his face or with his body language. He very clearly asked, "Can I go now?" His wife thought maybe he wanted to get up in his chair and she assured him that he could when I was done. I very soon realized he was talking about going to heaven, as many of our patients imply as going to as death approaches.

The ache in the pit of my stomach and my years caring for the dying heightened my awareness that my patient was probably and almost unbelievably just minutes from dying. His daughter-in-law had also recognized his very rapid decline and stayed close to her mother-in-law, who now also noticed a major change in her husband's condition. I gently and lovingly comforted my patient, his wife and family. I quietly explained to his wife what I thought was occurring as I noticed his color was becoming paler and he was becoming unresponsive to voice or touch. His breathing had become quieter and slower.

His wife wrapped her arms gently around him and repeatedly said, "I love you, I love you." The little dog was carried to the bedside and was abnormally quiet, yet somewhat shaky, as he attended to his loving owner.

Twenty minutes after eleven, forty minutes after my arrival, this loving man took his last, peaceful breath on earth. The only words that made much sense at that moment was that this man of faith entered Heaven when his church friends and pastor would have been in prayer, certainly praying for one of their own.

If my computer had not malfunctioned, if my first patient had not cancelled her visit, and if my second patient had been further from my last, I would not have been witness to such a holy coincidence. God puts us where we need to be, even though we may not be aware of or acknowledge it at the time.

The Dreamer

A family and a hospice team of caregivers have an opportunity to form a very strong bond with each other in the midst of their loved one dying. Michael Becker, a hospice volunteer, tells of such a bond:

Allen, 63 years young, was a carpenter by trade and a dreamer by volition. He was a devoted husband, father, and grandfather who took much pride and joy in celebrating each of those roles to the fullest. His enthusiasm for life was contagious and his positive attitude and determination were an inspiration to all who knew him.

Proof of Allen's boundless spirit became more evident following his 1999 diagnosis of pancreatic cancer.

Allen had run a small company outside of Philadelphia where he manufactured art supplies. He further honed his carpentry skills by sometimes building small furniture pieces. His diagnosis came not long after he sold the business and bought his dream home in Florida.

Given the grim prognosis of less than two years to live, Allen took an immediate pro-active role in his effort to fight the illness. He searched tirelessly on the Internet for the latest studies and treatments. Chemotherapy and radiation treatments would drain him physically, but never dampen his youthful spirit. He traveled 1300 miles to New York City's' Sloan-Kettering Cancer Treatment Center for hormone therapy. He simply refused to be defined by his illness and was rewarded with an amazing amount of energy. He and his wife, Sandy, would travel and he would continue to take on small projects around the house.

Ever the dreamer, Allen was not content and decided to take on a larger project. He purchased a Marine 'work-boat', which was part barge and part tugboat. It was a steel hulled craft and had no interior furnishings, save for the navigation equipment and a small stool bolted to the floor at the helm.

He purchased the boat in Norfolk, Virginia, and sailed it down the intra-coastal waterway to Jacksonville, and then down the St. Johns River to its final moorings in DeLand. Once the epic journey was complete, the task of transforming the craft into a beautiful, livable houseboat was undertaken. He fitted it with a living and sleeping area, as well as a galley and head (kitchen and bath). By all accounts, it was a beautiful vessel and an astounding accomplishment by a man who was in the midst of the battle of his life.

After necessity forced the sale of the houseboat, he was left wanting more. Without a second thought, he began drawing plans for another craft. This would be a modest eight-foot sailboat, which would also be equipped with a motor, as well as oars. He did months of research reading books, articles in magazines, and searched the Internet for all the information needed to build the small craft from the ground up. He had pages of drawings with accurate measurements and details.

By the time construction began, Allen's health had begun to deteriorate further and Hospice of Volusia/Flagler was called to help with medication and respite. Still the project went forward. The construction phase was undertaken in the back yard workshop, proudly dubbed *The Old Dixie Workshop*. Sandy would often escort him and watch as the vessel took shape, first the frame, then the bending of the lumber for the hull, which had to be incredibly precise. Sometimes the walk to the workshop would be exhausting, yet another task would be forged and the project came one step closer to completion.

Being ever the family man, Allen was thrilled to have his daughters participate in the project when they could. Allison was called on to put the final coat of paint on the vessel.

Once the craft was nearly complete, it was necessary to check for buoyancy. The only way to do that was to launch the boat in the nearby St. Johns River. Since Allen's health had taken a turn for the worse, this became a community project involving his friends, family, hospice volunteers and staff. A trailer was secured and a launch site picked just a mile and a half from his home.

On a crisp, beautiful Florida morning, the launching of *The Dreamer* became a happening. His friends and family watched and cheered as Allen, Sandy and two of his grandchildren sailed among the many other vessels strolling down the waterway. It was a day of celebration and laughter. It was a day of memorable sights and sounds. It was a day another dream came true.

Allen, given two years to live in 1999, passed away in 2007 just two weeks after the launch. He accomplished so much and inspired so many, and his legacy lives on in a handcrafted sailboat aptly named *The Dreamer*.

A Gift of Music

On occasion the care we provide our loved one is inadvertently a positive reflection on the care of another. Cliff Jackson shares his story:

My father died about a year ago from Congestive Heart Failure. He gradually stopped eating and then stopped taking water. My sister and I took turns sitting with him the last few days. I was with him the last night. I was playing a CD hour after hour called *Mender of Hearts,* which is harp music and a woman singing a beautiful, loving refrain. His actual passing was a very peaceful experience.

There was another woman a few doors down whose husband was in the same condition. However, while Dad was calm and peaceful, the other man was in agony. Nothing seemed to ease his pain and his wife and two grown children were understandably distraught.

A couple times during Dad's final night, the woman visited our room. I welcomed her in and she sat for a while. The woman said how blessed I was that Dad was so peaceful. She was so grateful to have a few minutes of the loving peacefulness in our room. I think it helped her go back and face the difficulty of her situation.

A little while later when Dad had died, she asked if it would be all right if she said her goodbye to Dad, which of course was fine. As she left our room, I gave her the *Mender of Hearts* CD. I stayed with Dad for a while and soon noticed the music was playing down the hall. I walked down the hall and noticed their room was quiet other than the soothing music. The woman and I made eye contact and tears began streaming down both our faces as she told me "he likes it, he's so peaceful." Giving and receiving, living and dying, and sharing love was the gift I gave and received.

One Tear

The time frame upon a patient's admission to hospice to their time of death can occur over a wide variance of time... from minutes to many months, or even a year or two. Hospice nurse Sally Swanson will lead us through a hospice admission with only minutes to spare:

As hospice nurses we see dying patients on a regular basis, sometimes many patients in the same day. In order to work for hospice one has to be very clear in their mind about how they feel about death and dying to help focus on the job at hand. Every so often we are reminded of why we do this job.

The winter season usually means that we get very busy. Living in an area where everyone wants to be in the South where it is warmer during the winter months means thousands of people flock to the region to escape the cold. We call them 'snow birds.' Hospitals are usually much fuller and staff is always looking for another empty bed to put another patient. The emergency rooms are full and many times hospital and potential hospice patients have been waiting overnight in the emergency room for that next available bed on one of the nursing units.

As supervisor of hospice admissions nurses, it is my job to assure that the nurses are doing their jobs well. Every so often I get the chance to do what I still love to do, see patients at the bedside. You can tell very quickly about a situation by looking at body language, reading facial expressions and listening to bits and pieces of conversations.

We often get calls to 'hurry' and come see a patient that is imminently dying. Those calls are hard for everyone for they mean that we are already too late. Not only is the patient acutely ill with maybe only a few hours to live, or sometimes just minutes, but the family is in crisis as well. Often hospital staff is grateful when we arrive for they are busy too and really don't have the time needed to work through these situations.

I learned a long time ago in hospice nursing to measure the value of our work not in days or months but by minutes. If we can make a difference for a few short moments then it is worth every minute of every day we do this job. I often hear people say, "life is short"; for us, that statement brings on a very special meaning.

Today was no exception as we received a call from the Emergency Room to see a patient who came to the ER with what would later be determined to be a massive stroke. Each new patient's story is unique to that individual and sometimes very sad. Each person has an entire life history that is quickly being told by the family in the few short minutes after we first meet.

Today's story was no exception. This one was an elderly gentleman who, according to the sons and daughters, was at home taking care of his wife who had some form of Alzheimer's dementia. Sometimes families leave many details out but give us enough to understand what has been happening in that person's life. According to the family and medical record, he had been 'found down' at home. What that means is that he had collapsed at home and was found on the floor by the Paramedics when they arrived.

The story goes on to say that this gentleman was caring for his wife who was now in a wheelchair at home. The wife wasn't able to call and let anyone know due to her condition so he didn't receive immediate attention. Fortunately for this family, they had regular visits from their church family. One of the church members, according to the story, became concerned, as they had not heard from the husband in a while. A visit was made to the home and the husband was found on the floor unresponsive. The family was called and wanted to call 911. Interestingly enough, it was reported that this gentleman had a *Do Not Resuscitate* paper signed by his doctor. However, when the time comes, many of us struggle with making a decision to not send someone to the hospital and so 911 does get called. The family asked the Paramedics to do everything they could. That means starting life support measures and transporting to the hospital.

When this gentleman arrived at the Emergency Room, he was placed on a respirator, as his condition was very grave. Further testing was done and it revealed a very large stroke. These types of family conferences are very hard as the news is not good and the outcome is usually very grim for the patient. After talking with the doctors, the family decided to honor this gentleman's wishes and *let* him go peacefully.

Now we all know how hard that kind of a decision is for families, as it means a loss to them and a big change in their lives without this person. Here is usually where hospice gets called to provide comfort and support. Families are devastated by the news and feel a volume of emotions. Sometimes anger, generally almost always an immediate sadness. This family, as many families do, finds the pain too much to bear and don't want to be there at the end. They graciously listened to our explanation of our hospice services, signed our paperwork, and then left the Emergency Room physically and emotionally exhausted.

The hard part of these cases is knowing the fact that this patient will die without family at his side. Don't get me wrong; we understand that the pain is too much to bear and that is why families sometimes can't do the *deathwatch,* as it is commonly called. But never the less, the end will come.

With these times, come those special moments. The hospice nurse who met with the family at first got all the paperwork signed, but couldn't stay as the next emergent call came for her to leave and talk to another distraught family. The nurse who would finish the admission hurried to get there so the patient hopefully wouldn't die without anyone at the bedside.

As I arrived to oversee her work it was obvious that the patient was very close to death. He had been removed from life support, at the family's request, and his breathing was now very shallow. He had a waxy look, which means his circulation was greatly impaired. The heart monitor showed a heart rate of somewhere around 28 and we knew the end was very close. I asked the hospice nurse if he had shown any movement or signs of responding and she said, 'I saw one tear.' My heart jumped to my throat and I thought how amazing it was that he was able to show us one sign that he was still here and somehow know the end was close. I tend to feel a vast amount of emotion at these times not knowing if he was crying because he couldn't say goodbye, or because he was sad to leave his elderly handicapped wife behind that he so lovingly cared for all this time, or for some other reason- just to let us know he was still here on earth.

You feel compelled at these times to stay at the bedside until the very end and we did, quietly holding his hand. Another hospice nurse walked in the room to see if we needed help and we said no that the angels were here. She said, "I think the angels have taken him already and they are gone." She said that she very often knows when the angels are here and she felt like they had already gone. The hair on the back of my neck stood up and we stood quietly for a moment, each of us with our own thoughts. I was grateful we could all be there together today with this gentleman feeling like, for one short moment, we made a difference in his life for the short time we were all together.

The hospice nurse at the bedside said to me, "I just couldn't leave him alone," and I knew she was right...we just couldn't leave him there alone to die by himself. He died peacefully that day with angels at his bedside and us just wanting to comfort him for his last few moments.

As we called the family to let them know he had just passed away peacefully, another frantic phone call came in to say there was another emergent admission of another imminently dying patient.

As I was driving home from work, late as usual, I felt compelled to say a prayer for this gentleman and his family as I often do for our hospice patients and their families. But my prayer was much more, for I not only asked for God to watch over this man who gave so much of his life to care for his wife, but for his family that had to make that agonizing decision today. I also prayed for myself. I thanked God for all the blessings he has given me in my life. For you see, I get to go home to my husband tonight and enjoy our time together for another day.

Goeff and Ivy - the Bedside Party!

Sweet Charity Hospice, located on the east coast of Spain, has been a saving grace for so many hospice patients and their loved ones since founded in 2004 by Martha Harlam. I stumbled upon *Sweet Charity Hospice* one day while searching on the Internet and after emailing Martha I sent her copies of our first books, *Dying with Joy and Sorrow* and *More Joy Than Sorrow.* Thus began a new and treasured friendship with Martha. I asked her if she had a story she would like to submit for this book from the other side of the Atlantic Ocean and, thankfully, she did. Here is Martha's story:

There are so many stories that could be added to the list of life and death chronicles that would fill out the pages of my hospice adventure. But one of the most moving and poignant stories of all is that of the final weeks and days of Geoff, up in the Urbinisation La Marina. This is a true story of love, passion and compassion for an unseperateable life together of 56 years.

Geoff and Ivy have lived in La Marina for nearly sixteen years. Their retirement in Spain was a source of joy and happiness. The sun filled years of blending in with the Spanish locals filled their lives with local Spanish traditions full of fiestas and daily cultural exchanges far beyond that of cold England. Ivy told me that there wasn't one day that they craved for "Fish and Chips" in Spain. Spain was Paradise on Earth for them. But that was all soon to change.

Goeff had been diagnosed this year with terminal cancer. The doctors at the hospital had basically sent him home to die with little or no provision of after care. At age 82, they packed him off in an ambulance with his blue hospital gown still on him, set him on his front porch and left him holding his clothes and personal belongings. If it had not been for his helpful neighbors, Ivy (80 years old) still doesn't know how she would have managed alone to get Geoff in the house and to his bed. It seems like a horrific description, an almost inhuman account, of what actually happened, but every word is true.

Ivy knew that she would need help coping with the end phase of Goeff's needs. This frail, little whisp of a woman was way in over her head. Goeff's needs were far more extensive than she alone would be able to cope with so she began calling support groups throughout the region. One that Ivy called turned out to be no help at all. They didn't even bother to answer her messages left on their answering machine. Another said they had no provision for home care needs at all. Yet another one came out to the house to read, play cards and Dominos with him but that is not what Ivy needed or wanted. "Is there no one that can help me CARE for my Goeff ?" The sixteen years of praise of the socio-economic policies of Spain were slowly being chipped away into a rubble of horrific nightmares.

Ivy made one last desperate phone call to the *Sweet Charity Hospice Fund.* Inside of one hour Head Nurse Gina Palmatuseck arrived at Ivy's door. Hope and help had arrived. Sweet Charity's policy is to always follow up with a home or hospital assesment. They might not be able to rescue all situations but you are never left in dispare to tackle your problems alone. Their policy is "Yes we can help you and if we can't then we work out a solution together."

Gina reported back to me and the very next day both Gina, Barbara and myself were at Ivy's side. Gina was in Goeff's bedroom making sure he was washed, comfortable and getting enough fluids. Meanwhile Barbara and I sat with Ivy listening to her stories of their past and attended to her questions about everyday care problems for both she and Goeff. We discussed everything from shopping needs, meals on wheels, pharmacy calls, cleaning, and visits from the Palliative Care Unit from the hospital social services. We even discussd the pending funeral arrangements. Ivy confided in us that both she and Goeff had donated their organs to the University Medical Hospital in Alicante. No funeral or clergy contact would be necessary. It was a total assement of Ivy and Geoff's needs on a very personal and compassionate level.

As the days went by and our visits became more regular we became a close knit family. One incident sticks out in my mind the most. Goeff was begining to loose his ability to speak his wishes but he could hear us and his mind was still as sharp as a tack. Ivy knew the end was near and we all sat at Goeff's bedside. Somehow Geoff made Gina realise that he was thirsty. But now was not the time to have water. Geoff wanted a sip of his favorite red wine.

And so it was! Gina propped him up against herself on pillows and we all joined Geoff and had a red wine party. This was a great day for Geoff. He was still calling the shots. Ivy made phone calls to update the family and we were with them right to the end. What a privilege.

Grandpa Saves the Day

Grandparents around the world have protected their grandbabies as long as time has been recorded. Grandparents have been deemed by some as the forgotten grievers and perhaps grandchildren also.

My twenty-three year old hospice patient shared in her grief, her love, and her loneliness for her deceased grandfather. She told me how he always understood her so well and so she wasn't surprised it was her grandfather that saved her day, years after his death. She explained, "I told my husband through my tears that I cannot do it any more. No more chemotherapy." Her latest treatments made her so sick that she told her husband it was impossible for her to have any quality of life any longer and the treatments were to stop.

Later that day, when alone and sobbing into her pillow, she sensed someone in the room with her. As she lifted her head from out of her pillow she saw her grandfather standing at the foot of her bed. Without any words spoken, he gently placed his hands on her feet which immediately initiated a very warm sensation that moved up her entire body. Miraculously, within twenty minutes her symptoms totally subsided and she was able to get out of bed and attend to her child and husband, which she hadn't been able to do for some time.

Many of our hospice patients have visions of those who have passed on before them, just like this granddaughter did. Another of my patients told me that for several days he had sensed angels around him as he sat in his recliner. He said that they gently bumped up against him. One angel placed a hand on his shoulder and he felt an immense warmth flood his body. He assured me he was on no medications, which some caregivers may say would explain what he felt. Without any doubt, I believed him. He died several days after sharing his angel story.

Hello Dan Blocker

Being a caregiver can be one of the most difficult emotional rides ever to be taken, especially if it involves placing your loved one in a facility. Karen Sutton's story portrays the ups and downs she experienced:

"Mr. Stack, who is that?"

"This is my daughter," my father beams at the aide walking alongside us down the hallway.

"And what's her name, Mr. Stack?" His blue eyes widen, momentarily confused and frightened as he looks over to me blankly.

"I'm Karen, Dad." I pat his arm comfortingly as we continue towards his room.

"He talks about you all the time," the aide tells me, as if to assure me that even though he doesn't remember my name anymore he remembers me. I don't need her kind reassurance. I already know that as his one constant, I am the light in a life that is becoming increasingly dimmer. It's both an honor and a terrible burden.

Like many others, I have recently had to make one of the hardest decisions of my life. Difficult decisions, it seems, have often been left to me- divorce, failing health, mental illness. So it was only natural that I would have to be the one to make the decision to place my father in an Assisted Living Facility/ALF for dementia.

My mother, long divorced from my father, accompanied me on the extremely depressing business of visiting ALFs, trying to choose one for my father. Together we walked up and down hallways of elderly residents, many pushing walkers or wheelchairs, some trailing oxygen machines beside them. We smiled and nodded countless hello's to people just happy to see another face, often thinking ours was one they knew. We watched them play games, knowing my father would not want to participate in them. Each room we looked at was different- some old and dingy, some cleaner and newer, large and small. Many had the faint smell of disinfectant and urine. But all had the smell of despair and finality.

Lunch has finished and the hallway is busy with patients in search of their rooms or sitting vacantly in the common room. A few talk animatedly as they walk through the hallways. My father is one of the lively ones. He greets most everyone as he passes them, occasionally stopping to chat, although for the most part what he is saying is unintelligible. He is rapidly losing the part of his brain that deals with comprehension and speech. The other patients don't seem to notice that he is not understandable. They smile or continue to stare blankly as he continues to proudly reintroduce me. "This is my daughter," he repeats to the same people I have met every week since he has come to live here.

His facility is small, with cozy rooms and open airy corridors. The rooms look out over a nicely landscaped inside courtyard accessible to all the patients from interior doors. This had been one of the deciding factors in choosing this place. I wanted my father to have access to the outdoors, to sit in the sun and be warm. It costs more monthly than he receives from his pension and Social Security and his small savings will dwindle quickly, but I've decided to cross that bridge when it comes. And it may not even come. His dementia is aggressive and he is already under hospice's care.

The day I decided on this facility my father sat next to me depressed and frightened. As he looked around at the fate about to become him, his voice broke. "Well, I guess this has to happen to just about everyone sooner or later," he stated resignedly to the administrator. "I guess I have no other choice." But he was clearly devastated and it took all my resolve to continue the admitting process. Used to the freedom of his own apartment, aided each day by a home health care worker who showered personal attention on him, this was going to be a prison for him. However, in this prison, I knew he would not forget meals, wander nights across dangerous streets in pursuit of a bottle of wine or leave his keys in the door, he sleeping inside, his cat forgotten and wandering alone outside.

At first, I came to visit him daily. Each time I would find him lying depressed on his bed waiting for me or agitatedly roaming the halls.

"Oh thank God you are here, please take me home with you," tears welled in his eyes as he pleaded with me. "I can't live here. What did I ever do to deserve this?"

The answer, of course, is nothing. Like almost all of us he has done both good and bad in his life. But he had never been evil or deviant or intentionally hurtful, just a fairly ordinary man of quick wit and large intelligence. This experience has left me even more confused about any divine master plan. I have worked hard to shore up my fragile belief that our lives have purpose, that each experience, especially painful ones, are about learning lessons, moving on, expanding our spirit. Can this be true if in the end we can't remember a thing?

Dad's constant pleas to me were heartbreaking. As I watched him decline physically and mentally at a much faster rate than ever before I wondered if it was the disease alone causing this or the fact that he had much less personal attention here than in his own home. I wondered constantly if I should have done something differently. It was as depressing and scary for me to look around at the other residents in various states of mental decline as it was for him. Was this my destiny too?

I decided I must put some space between his situation and myself. This was going to affect me detrimentally also if I didn't set some parameters. I began to limit my visits, keeping them regular but not as often. I actively tried to make peace with my decision, looking for all the reasons it was the correct one. I concentrated on staying in the present moment and not project this into some frightening future for myself.

My father's condition continues its precipitous decline. Not a large man to begin with, he has dropped thirty pounds in three months, mostly muscle weight. He has become incontinent. He is noticeably more disoriented, his memory regressing, his awareness of what is happening around him less. His speech is difficult to understand, often he uses the wrong words to try and convey his meaning. Sometimes he cannot remember to use his silverware and tries to eat with his fingers. He has become unable to figure out how to orient himself to sit down, often falling. After three months of living here and a change in medication he seems to have hit a plateau emotionally. He is fairly content, although not happy, most of the time. He still asks to come and stay with me, but it isn't the desperate, heartbreaking pleas of before.

Amazingly, he has a couple of girlfriends. Despite remains of lunch or dinner still apparent on his shirt, flakes of dandruff on his beard and jumbled, unintelligible speech, he is the resident Casanova. One of his girlfriends joins us now as we head toward Dad's room. As the three of us walk along the corridor to his room, both of them animatedly conversing with me, I nod and smile or shake my head. I hope that the occasional "yes" or "no", or "is that so" actually is a correct response to what they may be trying to say. Over the weeks of visiting Dad I have found that this strategy usually works. Mostly, I don't understand the gist of his conversation, but every once in a while he will have a brief time when his speech is clearly enunciated and understandable. These times are becoming less and less.

At the door to his room, I convince his girlfriend that we will see her later. Dad and I go in to watch TV. His ability to comprehend a story line has been gone a long time, but I always try to find a TV show or movie with familiar actors. My father is the published author of over twenty westerns, so I look first for an old western TV show or movie. Today, it is *Bonanza. The Ponderosa* fills the screen as Ben Cartwright, Little Joe and Hoss ride into view. As they dismount my father clearly exclaims, "Boy that Dan Blocker was a big man!" He may not remember my name today but I'm happy that for the moment he knows who Dan is.

Mama's Last Derby Roses

Birds, butterflies, dragonflies, rainbows, pets, angels, flowers… the list is much longer than this about how each has somehow touched those left behind during and after one's passing. Marie V. Sayre begins with her Mama's beautiful story that occurred while she and her brother cared for their mother:

It is said, "You can take a girl out of Kentucky, but you never take Kentucky out of the girl!" Mama was such a Kentuckian, born in Gravel Switch, Marion County in 1914. She was much loved and a great sport. She knew Kentucky basketball; she followed both the NCAA men's and women's collegiate tournaments as well as the Kentucky Derby contenders each year and also enjoyed her bourbon- Maker's over cracked ice with a twist.

It was my brother's ritual to give Mama a dozen roses at Derby time, which on occasion coincided with her May 5 birth date as it does this year, 2007. Mother's Day is frequently within another week. This year it falls on May 13 when her eldest great-grandson will make his First Communion in Plano, Texas.

In March of 2006, Mama's lung cancer had progressed to the stage whereby she elected to call Hospice of Volusia/Flagler rather than pursue further aggressive medical intervention. How fortunate for Mama, my brother and myself! With their concerned bedside care and psychological support, my brother and I were able to spend Mama's last weeks competing over the NCAA men's basketball tournament, talking about the early Kentucky Derby contenders and communicating with other family members and friends. As usual Mama won the NCAA 'picks!' Yes, the tradition continues!

The week before Easter, April 16, 2006, my brother came home with a dozen red roses and told Mama they were her Derby roses. I arranged the flowers in a vase at the end of her bed so she could enjoy them. The next morning, to my dismay, two of the stems had withered and bowed their heads. I checked the water level and all was normal. I turned the withered roses to the rear of the arrangement and concentrated on sharing Mama's moments of wakefulness.

The next morning two additional stems had withered and bowed their heads. Again I re-arranged the bouquet to place the bowed heads toward the rear. I had never seen fresh cut roses act like that unless they were out of water or bruised.

Mama received phone calls from Colorado, from Virginia, and from Kentucky. Her friends and neighbors were very loyal about checking on her comfort. On the third morning, two additional stems had withered and bowed their heads. As I was re-arranging and fretting over the quality of the bouquet with six bowed stems, the hospice nurse suggested that maybe Mama was gathering them to her and planned to take them with her. I had certainly never given that a thought!

We were expecting two of our cousins, her youngest niece and nephew, to visit from Virginia and New York. They were bringing his children, a great-nephew and a great-niece whom she had never met. Upon their arrival the next day, again two stems had withered and bowed their heads; eight were now bowed. Mama was resting very peacefully after focusing intently on her visitors, especially the children and their comments: one shared a family name with her, McDonald; the other associated her name with Rudolph's girlfriend, also named Clarice.

As we watched the bouquet on Saturday, two more stems withered and bowed their heads. Shortly before noon on Easter Sunday 2006, my brother sensed that he needed to check on Mama. As he looked in on her, he was alarmed by her stillness. He called to me. I slipped my hand behind her head and whispered: "Mama." Mama's eyelids fluttered and opened one last time. Then with a breathless little sigh, she left us just about noon; the last two roses were bowed. We think the hospice nurse had the best explanation about the roses. It is comforting to believe that Mama gathered and took her last Derby Roses with her.

An Unexpected Healing

There are many miracles that occur throughout our lives, whether we recognize and acknowledge it or not. When we think of miracles, most of us probably recall some of the great miracles Jesus and his disciples performed as recorded in the Bible. What we have considered luck or coincidence that has occurred in our life may have actually been a miracle. Here's my family's miracle I would like to share with you:

While in nursing school, I had the honor to practice my new care giving skills on a well-loved patient, my Grandfather Vincent. He resided in a nursing home and on occasion, when he was able, he would go to his home for several hours on a weekend. If I was home from college, I would go and help transfer Grandpa from his wheelchair to his bed, so he could take a short nap, and then back to his wheelchair. It was a tricky thing to do with me weighing in at 102 lbs. (which is definitely not what I weigh now) and Grandpa easily doubling my size. Believe it or not there is a safe way to transfer someone under these conditions. I have seen nearly all my patients' loved ones learn how. Allow me to regress a bit for the main gist of the story.

On the morning I left for my very first day of college devastating news struck the Fairchild family. My grandfather had a massive stroke and left him totally paralyzed on one side of his body, near mute, and understandably very depressed and withdrawn- nothing like the Grandpa I knew.

My Grandma's faith and belief in an all-powerful God gave her the assurance that the love of her life could be healed and so without a doubt she asked her church's pastor and the church's District Superintendent, who was also a pastor, to say prayers over Grandpa asking God to totally heal him from his severe disability.

Before the private prayer service, the minister spoke with my father Carlton, Grandma and Grandpa's second oldest son, and asked what he thought his mother's expectations were. My dad assured him that Grandma expected a total healing! With that in mind, a private prayer service was held with Grandpa, Grandma, Dad, the local pastor, and the District Superintendent present.

A miracle did happen but not the one Grandma expected. Grandpa was not healed physically but rather he was healed spiritually and emotionally as demonstrated when he often smiled and held his head up and joined in the camaraderie of his very large and extended family. He laughed sometimes with tears of joy as his belly shook like Jell-O, and he would join in conversation even though the only words he could speak were fewer than the fingers on his hands. He was grateful for every day of the ten years he lived thereafter with my Grandma visiting him nearly every day. Their six children all played an active role in his care giving. Grandpa had some down times just like we all do, but none would cause him deep depression like he had experienced before his miracle.

My father had never shared this story about Grandpa's private prayer service with anyone until recently, over thirty-five years after his healing. Dad is now 82, near the same age my Grandpa was when he died.

What I learned from this story, and I sincerely hope you do too, has been reinforced for multiple years through many of my patients and their families. There are different kinds of healing, physical, emotional, spiritual and mental, and we don't always get what we pray for... but sometimes what we get is far better than what we asked for.

A Miraculous Language

There are some condominiums on the east coast of Florida that require you to walk outside on their balconies or walkways to get to the front door. Of course, these doors my patients lie behind can be many floors above the pavement below. That is not always a welcome thing especially if there is a strong and cold wind coming off the ocean, which causes my already frightful knees to rattle even more. Nonetheless, my hospice visit on this particular day was to assist the caregivers and my patient, who were many floors above the pavement yet worth the hike.

Lilly's adult children were so relieved when I stepped through their doorway as they felt their mother was very close to dying and was uncertain as to what to expect and what to do. They told me their mother's native language was Spanish, which I know none, so I apologized for my lack of ability in communicating with her. They assured me that was not a concern at all. Another great story evolved.

After spending half her life in South America where she was born, Lilly moved to the United States. She spoke Spanish in her everyday household and learned just enough English so she could communicate some with those in her adopted country.

As Lilly approached dying, she became weaker and unfortunately took a tumble one day, injuring her hip. With no reasonable explanation, Lilly's preferred language suddenly changed from her native Spanish to speaking fluent English. As a result, what I thought would be a challenge in communicating with my hospice patient was not a challenge at all, for which her caregivers were very grateful for.

Kailynne- Our Miracle Girl

Miracles have already been addressed in this text but not through the eyes and heart of a child or her loving and so attentive caregiving mother. Together, Tammy and Kailynne Quartier have written their story:

Kailynne was an eleven-year-old girl, very outgoing, caring and a take-charge type of person. On May 17, 2006, she was diagnosed with a Stage III Anaplastic Astrocytoma tumor. This is an adult tumor that is very rare in children.

After Kailynne's diagnosis, she underwent cranial brain surgery at which time the doctor removed thirty percent of this deadly tumor. After this surgery she underwent two additional surgeries: a port was placed in her chest, which was used for medications, and a shunt was placed in her head that weeks later had to be revised. In between surgeries, Kailynne underwent several weeks of chemotherapy and radiation, along with MRIs (Magnetic Resonance Imaging which takes pictures of body organs).

Doctors told us it was time to make a move due to the fact Kailynne was not responding to the chemotherapy treatments and the tumor had grown. So in January 2007, we took Kailynne to Duke University Hospital in North Carolina and St. Jude Children's Hospital in Tennessee. After several treatments of chemotherapy at St. Jude, we returned to Florida in February.

On February 12, Kailynne was not feeling well and had to be hospitalized. Another MRI was done that indicated the tumor had grown double in size and that there was nothing else that could be done for her and she was going to die.

On the advice of the doctors we were told to call our other four children and family members in to say their good-byes. After hearing this from the doctor I shared with him that I believed the Holy Spirit or the Lord contacted me twice in my life and that both times it was about Kailynne. I was told that Kailynne was going to go over some big bumps in the road and that she was going to survive this.

I told the doctor that I believe what the Holy Spirit or the Lord had told me. I told him that we needed to find another protocol to put Kailynne on and that she was going to survive. The doctor just looked at me and said, "You have done more than most parents; there is nothing else."

I told the doctor that Kailynne was not ready to go and that we were not most parents. Therefore, the doctor said he would put Kailynne on a high dose of steroids so the pressure in the brain would go down enough for her to respond enough to say her good-byes.

While this was being done I spent every spare minute of my time on the phone calling doctors, looking for another protocol, and calling the churches asking for everyone to pray for Kailynne.

On February 14, the doctor released Kailynne to come home. Before we left the hospital, the doctor made arrangements for us to call Hospice because once she came off the high dose of steroids she would continually go down hill until she passed away.

On February 15, Kailynne began declining and by the next day she was not responding, eating or drinking and had to wear Depends. On that same day, her friends made arrangements for a company to fill our front yard with snow because Kailynne's dream was to see snow. She was propped up in the window so that she could see, even though she was unresponsive.

On February 18, hospice nurse Pat came to me and said, "Tammy, Kailynne's vitals signs are diminishing and she may have only a couple hours to live. After hearing this I had to be alone to speak with the Lord so I ran back to Kailynne's room and spoke very loudly to God telling him that if that was not Him or my Holy Spirit that talked to me then who was it and where were they taking my little girl.

During my talk with God, our church family began arriving and my son Justin walked into Kailynne's room and spoke to me calming me down as much as he could. I pulled myself together and went back to the living room to speak with my lovely Kailynne.

I told Kailynne how much she was loved by everyone and how her father and I would be fine if she was tired and wanted to go. I told her it was ok.

Well, the next morning Pat got off duty and another hospice nurse, Kate, arrived. At this time I told Kate that I believed Kailynne was thirsty. Kate advised me to give Kailynne little sips of Ensure through a needle-less syringe, which I did. When I placed the syringe tip in Kailynne's mouth she sucked the Ensure right out of the syringe. I was so excited at what just happened that I called Kate and Kailynne's Dad over to see what she had done. I filled the syringe again and placed it in her mouth and she sucked the Ensure from the syringe, while Kate and her Dad watched.

What happened next was a miracle!! Kailynne opened her eyes and told me that she loved me and wanted a grilled cheese sandwich. Well I made her that, cut it into small pieces, and she ate it. According to another hospice nurse, Jeanne, on this day they were suppose to start Kailynne on TPN (Total Parenteral Nutrition given intravenously) but now did not have to.

As Kailynne was waking up she told me that she believes she saw God and that he had some angels with him. Kailynne said God told her not to give up. On Thursday Kailynne was given another MRI. The results showed that the tumor had some shrinkage. Since that day Kailynne has regained her speech and some movement in her right hand and right leg.

Kailynne does not remember anything about the three days she was unresponsive. We believe Kailynne saw the Grand Physician of the world, God, and that he healed Kailynne and sent her back to us. She has since been placed on another protocol and the last MRI revealed more shrinkage of her tumor. We feel the above week was the biggest bump we will have to go over.

The doctor said he is amazed and that it was unbelievable that the tumor had shrunk. Kailynne is a strong believer in the Lord and the good Lord knows Kailynne has brought a whole lot of people closer to Him through her sickness and we believe that was His plan.

Since Kailynne woke up, the hospice nurses were no longer needed for 24/7 care. Her nurse Jeanne still comes once a week to check on Kailynne and Mae, her Certified Nursing Assistant, comes each day to help bathe her and paint her finger and toenails.

We have to remember that in trying times it is ok to rest but don't ever quit because you could be so close. Believe and you will receive.

Amen.

For five more months a miracle was performed through Kailynne by her blessing so many more lives with her presence until her death on July 16, 2007. For years to come, her story will continue to bless and inspire countless more.

A Child Remembers

A man introduced to me through a hospice co-worker was in my home servicing a piece of equipment. While working, he told me this story about his childhood miracle.

At near eighteen-months-old and able only to speak a few words, this little boy was deathly ill with spinal meningitis. In fact, his doctor told his family that only a few days would lapse before their son's death. The family called their priest to the bedside to administer the last rites, baptize him, and give him communion. Certainly, no one expected him to recognize or remember anything that occurred around him due to his young age and his grave condition.

To the amazement of everyone, in the few days that followed he awoke. What increased everyone's amazement even more was that this toddler began speaking in full sentences, even recalling in detail some of the events that had occurred as he lay dying.

When he became a teenager, he felt the need to clarify what really happened to him as a very young child as it was never openly discussed in his presence all those years. After telling his mother and grandmother what he recalled, they both confirmed that what he had heard snippets of and felt certain occurred years prior was very true.

Sing me a Song

Certain songs bring back lots of memories. Some songs recall happier times than others. I would bet that you could name a song now that holds a lot of meaning for you. One of my songs is "You are my Sunshine." That is the song I have sung to my two grandchildren since their births, and they can now sing-a-long with me.

On a Wednesday evening while visiting a patient new to hospice, we were having a great time conversing on all sorts of topics while addressing his health needs. Actually, I had just given him an enema and he felt so much better afterwards!

I try to never miss an opportunity, when I feel it is appropriate, to put a smile on my patient and caregiver's faces and an enema certainly wouldn't prevent my attempt on this occasion. So I told my very grateful patient that maybe this would be a perfect occasion to sing a happy song! And so he began singing, "You are my sunshine, my only sunshine..." I don't have to tell you how totally surprised I was that he chose that particular song out of the millions he could have chosen. What a holy coincidence! I shared with him that I sing that song to my grandchildren all the time. He just smiled.

I was hoping that I would have the opportunity to visit him and his wife again soon. However, he died four days later. I was so thankful I got at least one chance to share in their sunshine.

My next visit wasn't so enjoyable and certainly singing was not appropriate but a hospice chaplain visit was.

Daniel was in his 90's, his wife in her 80's. He was ready to die but she wasn't ready to release him. Her denial, anger, and bitterness would be reflected onto numerous caregivers and family who did realize that Daniel didn't have the stamina nor health to endure much more. I offered a chaplain in hopes that would bring them some comfort and closure but she adamantly refused, as that would "only make things worse." Then she inadvertently showed me why she may have felt so angry and bitter. With a near-silent whisper, so Dan wouldn't hear, she pointed a finger down toward the floor and said that's where she expected they would go. Then pointing upward she said, "I doubt if we will go there."

The Creativity of Veterans

After stepping up the weather beaten ramp to my patient's front door, I noticed what I thought was a typical recliner sitting on the front porch. Just as I stepped inside the home I knew I was about to enter a land of laughter and cheer despite the signs of illness that filled the home.

Vietnam heroes with tattoos and burly beards were attending to one of their own as he lay dying on this Memorial Day weekend. These heroes were there to ensure their buddy could join in the festivities on the lawn for what each recognized would be their last celebration together.

I needlessly voiced my concern over the comfort of my frail patient sitting for hours in his wheelchair outside. Then I was asked to look closer to the recliner I had passed on my way in- the one with a scrap metal base, four heavy-duty wheels attached underneath, and a truck dolly strapped to the bulk of it. These heroes were the ultimate caregivers and creators of comfort for one of their own. I salute you all! Thank you for providing me the freedom that many do not have.

A Miracle in Germany

Rev BJ Bishop has a very blessed relationship with God and always rejoices over His miracles, big and small. Her compassion, joy, and attentiveness to what He wants her to do is explained best by BJ:

My latest encounter with death happened last month. My friend Annalise, who visits us yearly in New Smyrna Beach, Florida, e-mailed me from her home in Germany to let me know she was terminal with cancer. She was so sorry she couldn't say good-bye in person. I talked with my husband Terry and knew that we had to go. So we left for Germany within a week with plans to stay for a week. That was the best listening to my heart I have ever done.

No one would talk to my dear friend about her impending death. Instead, they pretended it was not real. My role was to bring it out in the open, which I did, and you could almost hear the sigh of relief. She was so grateful that I forced her husband to quit hiding from her, and not facing or talking to her or taking her out anywhere. He also hadn't said he loved her in years but he did then.

I took her a copy of the book *Death and Dying*, plus some comforting music. She was so happy with them all. I prayed for God to be with me as it was all so delicate...and He was.

She wanted to have as much of life as she could so we all decided to go out for dinner. As we were leaving, she said she forgot her medicine so she went back in the house to get it. I, of course, said I would get it but she said, "No." I said, " I will go with you." She said, "No." Spirit told me not to move, but let her go. I stood as if frozen.

She came back and as she got closer to me she fell flat on her face. Her false teeth flew out and blood was everywhere. I felt so bad and Terry thought they would feel we had caused this by taking her out.

The ambulance came but she wouldn't stay in the hospital because we were there. A miracle happened when the two of them hugged and he again told her how much he loved her.

The next day we had her teeth glued and there were no bruises on her face!! If you could have seen how she fell flat on her face, you wouldn't have believed that was possible. We actually went to dinner the next night and she enjoyed her meal.

What looked like something bad was just God clearing the way. The accident gave her husband a chance to show his love and me to see God at work once again. Life is so much more than what we can imagine. I thank God when the curtain is pulled back of our awareness and we can get a glimpse of what *is* real.

She died two days ago and it was peaceful. I still can't put the miracle into words well. The best gift I have given myself was listening to my heart and dropping everything and going to Germany when I did. I am so grateful to have the husband I do also. God is only good!

Roger's Rainbow

Caregivers often say to me that they don't know how I can do my job, caring for the dying all the time. My response is always the same, "My job is easy compared to yours as a full-time caregiver because I get to leave after my visit is completed, while you stay behind." I believe the hardest thing, physically and emotionally, that anyone will ever do is be a caregiver for their loved one who is dying. Yet, what an honor to be the chosen one. You better get a Kleenex while reading this beautiful story told by a loving, caregiving mother, Florence Childress, about her son:

I am writing to thank hospice for all they have done for my beloved son, Roger, and what they are now doing for me. I was not aware fully of the wonderful service that hospice provides, not only to the patient but also to the family members and caregivers. They are all so kind and compassionate. Roger taught us so much during his illness- he wanted to know exactly what was happening each step of the way. The nurses were so patient and with gentleness explained everything to him. I don't know of any other organization that is as helpful with not only the patient but also with all those involved. I believe it takes a special type of person to tend to those who are terminally ill and their family members. We have been so fortunate to have their support and care. They are truly angels, here on earth.

Now I would like to tell you about Roger and the special rainbow he sent to me. It was ten years this past June 24, 2007 that my son Roger died, having a rare type of cancer.

It was cancer of the bile duct. He was 54 years old and had everything to live for: a lovely wife, beautiful home, a great job as a counselor, and his own airplane. Roger loved flying and had his license to teach flying which he did on his days off. I only wish that it had been me that died instead of him. Here I am an old lady now, my life is at its end and his was just beginning and he so wanted to live.

During the last months of his illness and life, we spent many hours together. I would read to him and we would have meaningful talks, getting to know each other better. Living so far apart, Roger in Oregon and me in Florida, we didn't get to visit very often. Many times we talked about God and religion and heaven. I asked him to please, please send me a rainbow after his life was ended here, if he could, to let me know he was happy and okay. Well, bless his heart, he did just that.

After he passed away, June 24, 1997, I returned to Florida. Late Saturday evening I was so tired that the next day I stayed home and rested most of the day. Monday a.m. I went to breakfast at a café on the beach. Two ladies were sitting at the table next to me...they were talking about a rainbow. I went over and asked them when they had seen it and they said "yesterday" (Sunday). They said it was beautiful. I told them why I was interested and we all started to cry. I was so sorry I had not seen it for I had been resting. Then I asked Roger if he could and would send a rainbow soon. Well, that Friday as I got out of the car from eating dinner, I looked up to the sky and there was my rainbow!! Thank you, Roger.

I don't know where the years went. They passed so fast. It seems like just a short time ago that Roger was a baby in my arms. He was such a good little boy. There are so many things that I remember about him. He was always so concerned about me and everyone else. Many times when I was upset he would cheer me up. One time when I had been crying and was very upset, he said, "Mother, don't cry. God will take care of us." He gave me a big hug and kiss. That is one of my most precious moments with him. He was only five years old at the time.

When Roger was two, he had whooping cough and the doctor came to the house several times to give him Penicillin (it was new at that time). He asked me if he could cry that time, for I had always told him boys don't cry. (I now know that was wrong of me.) I so wanted him to be strong and grow up and be a good man.

After graduating from high school, Roger joined the Air Force. It was during this time when he began taking flying lessons and he obtained his pilot's license.

Roger was busy with work and flying but lacked a life partner. He met Debbie, his future wife, not long after moving to Portland in 1978. In 1983 they married. His family in Florida always hoped he would return to the area once he retired. Unfortunately, this was not to be.

In 1993 Roger was diagnosed with cancer of the bile duct. After surgery, he seemed to be doing okay. Then in 1996 the cancer returned. Again, he had surgery and was given about one year to live. His sisters, Gerri and Brenda, and I went to Vancouver (where Roger and Debbie were then living) to be with him. During the years he lived in Portland and Vancouver, we had all been out there to visit, but naturally not often enough.

Roger was always a comfort to me, even in his dying days. No one could have had a better son. I am grateful I was able to be with him the last three months of his life. I am most grateful that I was chosen to be his mother. I was blessed to have had Roger for the years that I did.

During his illness, he was fortunate to have the help of the hospice in Oregon. We all handle situations differently. Roger wanted everyone to feel at ease around him. He enjoyed having a house full of people around, family, friends, and co-workers. His sisters flew out three different times in those last three months and were able to re-connect after being so far apart for so long. It was a time of deep and heartfelt conversation…lots of hugs, laughing, crying and loving.

Now here it is, ten years later, and I'm under hospice care. How fortunate I am to have such caring individuals help me and my family through this part of my life's journey. Each one in their own way has been such a comfort.

I wrote most of this three years after Roger's death. It has now been ten years. I want to let people know that with God's help and work you can reach your goals even through difficult times. I am so thankful to God and to hospice for all they have done and are doing for my family and me.

A Young Mother

Darylnn Whiting, a hospice volunteer for nearly nine years, dedicates her story to the memory of a courageous young mother, who was a hospice patient, and to her loving family:

One warm summer day I was chitchatting with a fellow employee after a day of work in the Hospice Care Center. As we exited the building, I noticed a young lady sitting in a wheelchair just watching everyone pass her by. I looked at my co-worker and I said, 'I just have to say hello.' This is where our journey begins.

As I started walking back to this patient, I introduced myself and I asked her name. I also told her that I noticed she liked to sit outside and that I could bring her outside on my lunch break. She told me that she really just wanted someone to talk to. I told her that would be just fine and that I would see her that very next day.

Over the next couple of weeks we spent every lunch together whether I was working or not and we had wonderful talks. Our talks did not consist of dying, instead we talked about love, healing, family, God and anything and everything she wanted to talk about. I am not sure if I ever really said much, but just enjoyed listening to all of her stories of her young life, her caring mother, her 4-year-old son, and all of her extended family. I found myself really looking forward to each visit so we could laugh and cry and be afraid together of what may come.

This patient wanted to go home and continue to try and take care of her son and heal. On the day of her departure from the Hospice Care Center, I was upstairs working and all of a sudden I looked up and this patient was in my doorway. The Certified Nursing Assistant/CNA brought her upstairs in her wheelchair to say goodbye and take pictures. We shared more laughter and then the CNA and I helped get her into her mother's car for her ride home.

After this patient was not able to stay at home, she was placed in a nursing home very close to her family's home. I visited her a few times during her stay there and even though her disease had made her much weaker and pain had started taking its toll she shared more stories of her life and deep love for her son and family.

As her disease progressed and her pain needed more management she was transported back to the Care Center late one evening. The next morning I rushed to see my friend and we embraced tightly. Even though our talks were of healing and living, our eyes were telling a different story- a story of a 29-year-old dying woman with a 4-year-old child she would leave behind.

Upon her arrival back to the Care Center, the CNA caring for this patient had realized that her *reaching and grabbing* was her need to be held. So with the help of a couple wonderful hospice staff members they helped me get into her bed. She was only 68 pounds now, extremely frail, and even the slightest movement was painful for her. As she nestled her head on my chest, she grabbed me around the waist. I told her I would not leave her alone and for the next few hours I held her like a mother would hold a child so she could feel safe and rest in my arms. This patient fought to stay alive and did so for yet another night.

Upon arrival for work the next morning I went to visit her room. The hospice nurse was in the hallway and said that the patient needed a hug from me. I entered the room and noted she was still fighting for every breath and the look in her eyes was of fear and suffering. I bent down to hug this patient, looked into her eyes and told her that I would only be upstairs and that I would be back to check on her at lunchtime. I also told her that she needed to find a safe place and hide within herself. She nodded *yes* to me and I told her it was okay to hide from the pain.

With a heavy heart, I went upstairs to work. Then a couple of hours later I received a phone call. They said that this patient was not doing well and asked if I could come downstairs to be with her. (I have asked many people which special staff member called me that morning and to this day no one knows who made the call to me.)

I remember hanging up the phone and making my way downstairs. I would have to describe the feeling as being somewhat numb and walking through fog, not really hearing anything around me, just my own breathing. As I walked in this patient's room, we made eye contact and I let her know that I was there and would not leave her. I held her hand and just stayed right at her bedside.

When her nurse came back in the room she informed me the patient's mother had been called and she was on the way to the Care Center. With her nurse on one side and me on the other, we held her and when I knew she just could not hang on any longer I gently rubbed my thumb on her forehead and looked into her eyes. I told her that her Mommy was on the way and that her Mommy loved her very much. I told her it was time to fly away and she took her last breath. The nurse and I stayed right at her bedside and when her mother arrived I eased back and let her mother hold her baby girl. I then exited the room and the wonderful Care Center staff, along with the help of a chaplain, cared for this grieving mother that had just lost her child.

Elvie

While a patient is receiving hospice care in a nursing home or assisted living facility, they continue to receive care and attention from the staff who have attended to their daily needs for perhaps months or years. In fact, these patients become like family to the staff members and sometimes are the only so-called family their patients have. Bob Ellenberg's story beautifully portrays this bond:

Everyone at the nursing home, the hospice workers, the nurses, the aides, my patient's sons, and myself kept waiting for Elvie to take her last breath. She frequently looked at me, her friend and social worker, with questioning, painful eyes asking the words, "When will it come?" I shared the little I know about dying, telling her she's been given a long time to get ready.

A few months before her last breath, she went through a frightful period, admitting she was very afraid of what was to come. I tried to reassure her it was going to be okay by saying, "You've led a good life, raised four good sons, none of us are perfect, otherwise we wouldn't be in this life. It is our ground for learning."

In her weak, thin voice, trying to put on a smile of confidence, she asked, "Do you really think so?"

"Yes, I think so, Elvie, and everyone else that knows you thinks so, too."

Elvie has been mostly in bed during all this time. Until recently, she had been still continent, getting up on her own and using a potty chair next to her bed, then she had her first fall. Now she pulls the call light asking for help to take the three steps to the potty.

At some point she developed liver cancer that metastasized to her intestines. This put her into a frightful state as she began to claim the down side of her manic-depressive condition, although never losing her friendly nature. The cancer grew until she needed surgery, having a large portion of her liver and part of her intestine removed. With so much of her vital organs gone, it seemed only a short time before she passed.

After two months recovery, the oncologists recommended extensive radiation therapy. I was dubious about putting her through all this, especially the order for once a week treatment for forty-eight weeks. I had seen others go through extensive treatments when all seemed hopeless but she didn't know what else to do. I held my thoughts, as did the other doubting staff. We supported her in what she believed would give her more time on this planet, which it did, but was it worthwhile.

She followed the doctor's prescription but after three months of treatments she made her own decision to stop treatments. Unfortunately, the surgery and the radiation weakened her so that she became a bed patient but still maintained her friendly demeanor.

A few months after her surgery, I came to work one morning and was told Elvie was having an excruciating toothache. I was asked to get her to a dentist. I called the college dental clinic and was told they were closed for Christmas break but a skeleton staff would see her. It's usually impossible to get any one in on short notice and took this to mean it was right. Also, getting her a ride from the transport company without calling one day ahead for an appointment gave me further confirmation of the forces at work.

I didn't usually accompany residents to dental appointments but Elvie was special. I followed the transporting van to the hospital.

I assured her I would be by her side through it all, whatever that might be. My friend was sick and weak already. The dentist did his exam, found the tooth that needed to be extracted, but due to its crumbly condition it splintered leaving a jagged part sticking out of the gums.

When the jagged tooth was finally out after a very distressing experience and she was rested, I eased her into my car and drove her back to the home. For many months after, I felt responsible for a further deterioration of her demeanor, as she was even more lethargic, reticent, never wanting to get out of bed.

Elvie continued on for over a year post-dental procedure. In her final days she was getting smaller and smaller as she ate less and less, her abdomen swelling as the cancer returned, a tumor making itself a prominent feature of her body.

I was hard on myself when I'd get busy and for a day or two not find time to visit her, or sometimes even forget she was there, being absorbed in the lives of so many others.

Elvie continued on, barely breathing, barely able to do anything, now unable to get to the bedside commode. When her son was visiting from New Mexico, she was semi-alert and told him in no uncertain terms, "I'm not going. The cancer will stop." She still had not made peace with this life and struggled with the after life. I thought of all our talks and the reassurance she received from the hospice staff and me about the blessings she will receive, but yet was uncertain.

Two days before Elvie died I went to see her and as usual she was sleeping. A soft kiss to her forehead was enough to awaken her. She barely opened her eyes, looked up at me, smiled and didn't say anything, just looked for a moment or two. I simply said, "No more words." She shook her head *no* and closed her eyes. She died at 6:00a.m, a little before my morning meditation when I was asking God, or myself, if I can leave my job before she dies.

Spreading Joy and Love

The love we have for each other transcends life and death. Ann Waris portrays her family's love beautifully:

Of my nine siblings, my sister Geneva was my favorite. During my first year of life, Mom suffered from severe depression and most of my care was left to Geneva, age 17, at the time. I often lovingly referred to her as my sister, my mother. A year after I was born, she got married. My mother said I cried almost every waking moment for days after she left and moped around the house for weeks thereafter.

But Geneva didn't abandon me—us. She visited us almost every weekend. Every time my mother would allow it, she'd take me to spend a few days with her. After I was old enough to remember, I could hardly wait from one visit to another to spend time with her husband Edward and her. They were cheerful, funny and wonderful. They rolled out the welcome mat to all their friends and loved ones and showered them with love. All their guests were bound to have a good time. That never changed. Their home was filled with laughter and good cheer.

In 1979, her doctor diagnosed her as having cancer of the spine. He gave her only weeks to live. We were devastated. I had lost Mom when I was twenty-three and, to me, it felt as if I were losing my mother all over again.

The only one who didn't appear to be daunted by the unfortunate news was my sister herself. She said she wasn't quite ready to die and determined that she wasn't going to go so quickly, without warning. She lived six more years. During those years, she was the one who kept everyone else cheered up. She would allow no sadness over her condition from any of us, and that was that! When she lost her hair, she laughed. "My head looks like a shiny apple."

Loved by so many, her house was like grand central station with visitors coming and going, but that was her wish. Her life had always been filled with people and she had no intention of changing it. Visitors never seemed to tire her, but rather she appeared to thrive on their company.

Then came the time when she could no longer remain at home. But did that get her down? Not in the least. In the hospital, she was the same sister I had known all my life, making everybody laugh and reminding them of special moments they had spent with her throughout the years. No one could remain sad around her for long. She treated the hospital personnel the same way, spreading cheer around. They loved her.

Hours before she died, she said that she was ready. Her face was a picture of serenity. Though she must have been suffering horrendous pain, she never mentioned it. Obviously sensing the time was near, she hugged each of us goodbye and told us that she wasn't really leaving us, just going to visit with God for awhile until we decided to come and join her. She died with a smile on her face.

Understanding Pain

Since birth we have listened to adult conversations and been involved in our family's activities that most likely included discussions and/or activities relating to death and dying. Our comprehension of what dying is about, what behavior and responses are expected, the language used in relating to death, the rituals performed, and the values placed on the deceased slowly evolved. If we were raised not to fear death or dying but to understand it and maybe even embrace it then as adults we just may have obtained a mature concept of death.

Realistically, our mature concept of death is liable to be fleeting if events in our final days or weeks of life cause us untoward concerns or anxiety. Let us begin with what the majority of my end-of-life class attendees, my patients, and their care givers have told me is their greatest concern: uncontrolled pain. So I assume pain is probably what you would have also answered. Whether we have pain that is acute or suddenly occurring, or if we have pain that is chronic or long-standing, we all want it at a level we can easily tolerate, but understandably we would prefer none at all.

To best understand how pain can be anticipated and then controlled, I am using two scenarios that occurred with my hospice patients during the same weekend. This first scenario certainly and sadly could have been prevented.

Scenario #1: Lee has liver cancer and is cared for by his wife in their home. He has been a hospice patient for five days. His strength in providing his own physical care, administering the medications his physician ordered to control his symptoms, and voicing his needs has waned as he quickly approaches death. So now he must rely on his bride of fifty-five years to provide him his medications and daily care, as well as anticipate any unmet needs. She was not aware of Lee's medication routine before his decline and so consequently does not understand the importance of Lee receiving his medications on a regular basis. She also has concerns that Lee may be over sedated, not realizing that his sleepiness is due more to his decline in health and approaching death than due to his medications.

A fear some hospice patients or their caregivers may have is a drug addiction or dependence on pain medicines. That is not an issue with hospice patients. Their medication doses are ordered by their physician without the intent to hasten one's death or cause an overdose. Each medicine plays a significant role in providing a peaceful and comfortable quality of life at the end of life.

While providing care for Lee who was minimally responsive, I needed to gently reposition him to his side. During this brief moment of movement, Lee severely grimaced, moaned loudly and stiffened his body, indicating he was in great pain. Because his wife was present and observed Lee's very painful condition, a teaching-moment occurred and she quickly realized her error in judgment, so I thought.

With emotional support, end-of-life education, and stressing the importance of Lee receiving his medications, his wife decided to administer his medication while I was present and the pain crisis was soon resolved during this visit. She voiced the need for pain control and her understanding that the medications are normal doses, prescribed by their family doctor, and are not to hasten Lee's death, but rather he would pass on his own time. She assured me she would administer Lee's medications every four hours, like he took them on his own, and if she had any questions or concerns she would call hospice 24/7. Lee was very comfortable by the end of my visit and I informed them both that I would visit again the next day, or sooner if needed.

Very *unfortunately* for Lee, when I returned nearly twenty-six hours later, I discovered that his last dose of pain medication was when I visited the day prior! His wife had been awake with him all night and she stated she "was exhausted" and didn't know what to do. He very obviously was having another pain crisis and was extremely restless due to his uncontrolled pain, and perhaps imminent death.

Fortunately, their son who lived out of state had arrived just hours prior to my visit and stated he would gladly assist with his father's care and medication needs. So Lee's care needs as death approached and his medications were reviewed again with his wife and now his son, with both voicing understanding of all. There was still some reluctance on the wife's part that medications needed to be given regularly and she was adamant that their son not be overly involved in his father's care.

My heart was literally breaking for Lee. I offered his wife nurses to remain in the home to provide extra care and assist her, plus I discussed the availability of the Hospice Care Center for Lee, which she said she had considered the week prior. She refused both. I offered a hospice chaplain and a social worker to provide more comfort and support to her husband, their son and to her but she adamantly refused further assistance. Then she says, "He's not going to die and I don't want to talk about it." Her denial of Lee's approaching death was all she could focus on.

My awareness of this elderly lady not being in the best of health physically or emotionally is also my concern. Her failure to provide intimate care for her husband is not because she doesn't want to but simply because she is physically unable. Her anxiety over his possible death has escalated. She does not want her husband to die. He is her best friend and her life.

However, I am also aware that Lee has his own concerns. It is not only pain he must contend with but he may also have some anxieties regarding his approaching death. He may need an opportunity for closure and to complete some unfinished business his wife may not be aware of. Unfortunately, his wife would not allow any discussion from any member of the hospice team to discuss such anxieties and lack of closure on this day.

Lee died three days later. I do not know how this true story ended because his regularly scheduled nurse attended to him upon his death. I fervently prayed until then that he would have a peaceful and pain-free passing.

Scenario #2: Thomas has had ups and downs with his prostate cancer but one thing he has managed very well is his control of his pain. Five days ago he was admitted to hospice. He was already receiving pain medicine that he took every twelve hours, which is a long lasting or time-released medication. This pill controls his pain very well. Tom also has a pain medicine he can take every four hours if his long acting medication isn't working as well, which he notices especially when he performs more activities around the house.

Tom's wife recognizes that he is sleepier when he has to take extra pain medicine but she is always able to easily awaken him if it is time to take a pill or an unexpected visitor drops in. His wife is aware of his medication schedule and needs and is very grateful for his pain control. His hospice nurse had informed Tom and his wife that he may need to have his doctor increase his medication dose in the future as it is common to develop a tolerance to a lower dose and so it may not be quite as effective. Together they will monitor closely for that need.

Tom died very peacefully three days after my visit, without pain or other symptoms hindering him, as his wife carefully monitored his need for medications and administered each when appropriate. She lovingly held him when he passed on to the heavenly life they both anticipated.

Medicine and Misunderstandings

Patients in the United States are often under treated for pain according to a report by *The National Foundation for the Treatment of Pain*. As one who has worked for years in hospitals and visit them regularly, plus I know a large handful of friends who battle chronic pain, I would have to agree. However, I believe pain control is of utmost importance in caring for hospice patients and hospice staff does a superb job in managing pain, and certainly other symptoms. The medicines prescribed are to provide comfort and improve one's quality of life at the end-of-life.

Drowning in Morphine was a headline in an e-mail I got several years ago that made my blood boil. Education is a critical component to ensure our patients and families feel comfortable in administering prescribed medications. Here is an example: one of our patient's family members who had just arrived from out of town was so sure we were *killing* his loved one with Morphine, prescribed for her cancer pain, that he decided to withhold his mother's medicine. Within eight hours, she had a pain crisis that was off the charts. Of course, it took some more time to get her back to a tolerable level of pain and anxiety control. He felt certain her medicine is what caused her physical decline and not the fact she was approaching death.

Another example: I visited a chronic smoker/lung patient on a Saturday who was in severe respiratory distress. She became confused and forgot to take her Morphine, which she did not need for pain control but rather to ease her breathing. Her caregiver did not realize her medicine had not been taken but soon discovered she had not. Even when my patient was receiving around-the-clock Morphine, she was awake and alert and able to carry on a normal conversation without any shortness of breath.

Just several hours later, as I was nearing the end of my Sunday hospice visits, I visited a gentleman who was just hours from death. When I entered his home I knew it was wrapped in love by the butterflies that dangled from the top of the curtains near his bed, the Bible on the end table, the portrait of Jesus on the wall, and his very loving family attending to his needs. Each voiced concerns that my patient acted painful through his moaning and grimacing, and he appeared anxious, restless, and "jittery". His wife reported that for years all he was used to taking was an occasional Tylenol, so his sudden change in his condition was of concern. She also reported he was no longer able to swallow pills or liquids.

Because of an increased risk of aspiration in patients approaching death and a decrease in ability to swallow pills, a doctor can order medicine to be administered in liquid, suppository, or topical form. Liquid Morphine was already in my patient's home with the anticipation that it may be needed. After explaining the drug's purpose to my patient, who gave me a squeeze with his hand indicating he understood, and to his family, I was given permission to give some Morphine. I administered drops in his mouth, which did not cause him to choke. Over the next thirty minutes, he settled to a much calmer state and was still able to provide some interaction with his family, even though he was only hours from death.

Toward the end of my visit, his daughter voiced a request, "You are obviously a Christian woman; would you mind if we all have a word of prayer at Dad's bedside?" And so we did as a calm settled over my patient and his very loving family. There is no better way to end my day.

Death on the Other Side of the World

Pain is not always controlled here or on the far side of the globe. I was sadly reminded of that when I visited Indonesia in July 2006 with my brother, Gary. During a conversation with one of the gentlemen we had met, I asked him if there was a hospice in the area. He had never heard the term hospice. So I asked him where most people die. He said his mother had just recently died in their extended family home because they couldn't afford the hospital. He said that in order to stay in the hospital you must pay for your care and medicine on a daily basis or you will be discharged home. That is difficult to do when the average middle class salary in this area of Indonesia is $3/day. He told me his elderly mother was in severe pain until her last breath, with her family at her side. Are we a blessed country or what?

Asking for Hospice

Hospice care is available in many areas across our nation so there is probably one in your area. Your doctor will know where one is, they may be listed in your phone book, or you can research the numerous resources available on the Internet, and some are referenced in the back of this book.

To receive hospice care, an order must be obtained from one's doctor who anticipates a life expectancy of six months or less. If you feel you or your loved one is in need of hospice care, you can call a hospice organization yourself to get more information and they will make the appropriate doctor contacts or you can ask your physician yourself.

Most insurance companies provide hospice coverage; also Medicare and/or Medicaid may be available. A hospice team member will assist you with monetary concerns. No one should ever be turned away from hospice due to lack of finances. Memorial funds are often available to assist those who have insufficient funds.

When we talk about hospice care and end-of-life decisions, we must address the need for Advance Directives and legal documents that stipulate what our wishes are regarding health care, estate distribution, and who we wish to advocate for us if we are no longer able. Our next chapter addresses these concerns and, as difficult as it may be, it is best to make such decisions before others are required to make them for you.

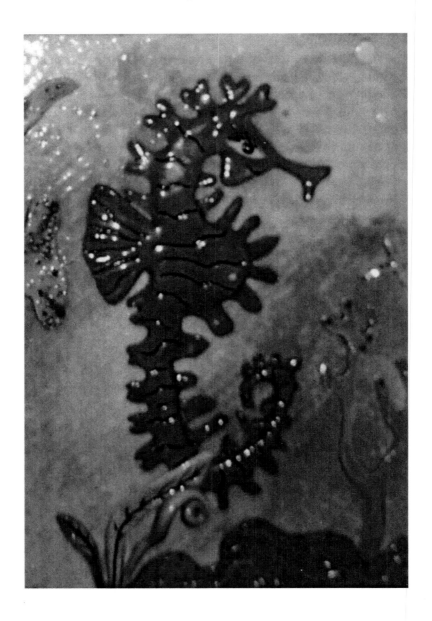

The Miracle Seahorse- story pg. 16

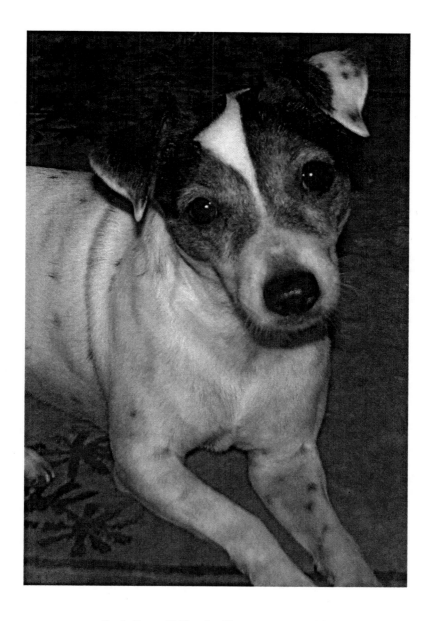

Jack Russell Terrier Dog- story pg. 18
Photo courtesy of Ann Horn

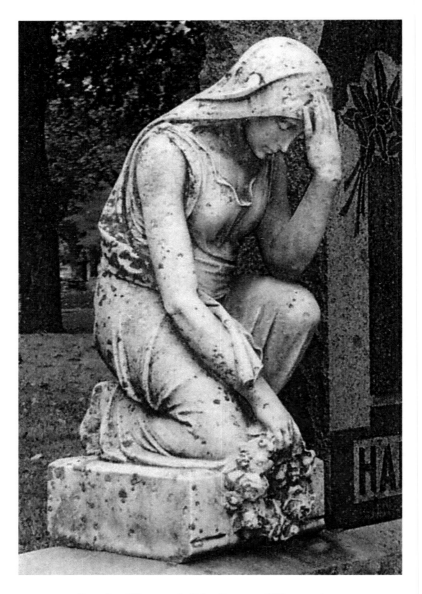

Praying Woman in Manitowoc, WI cemetery

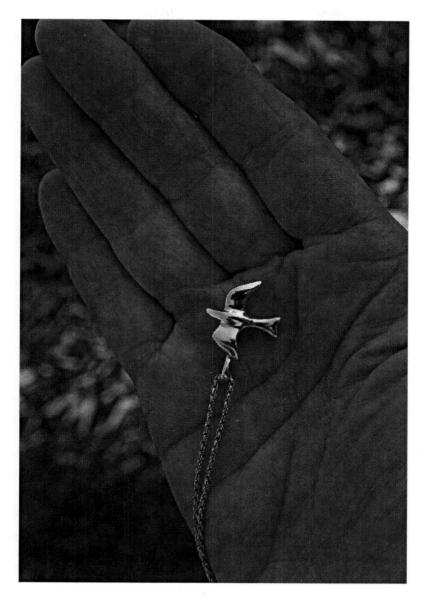

Mum's Dove Necklace with Ashes enclosed
Photo courtesy of Barbara and Warren Graham

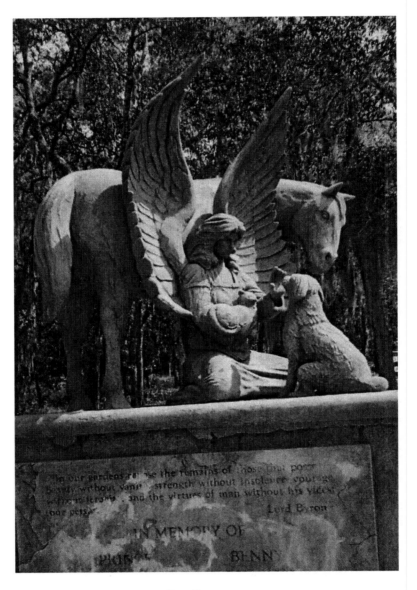

Pet Cemetery
Rt. 441, North of Ocala, FL

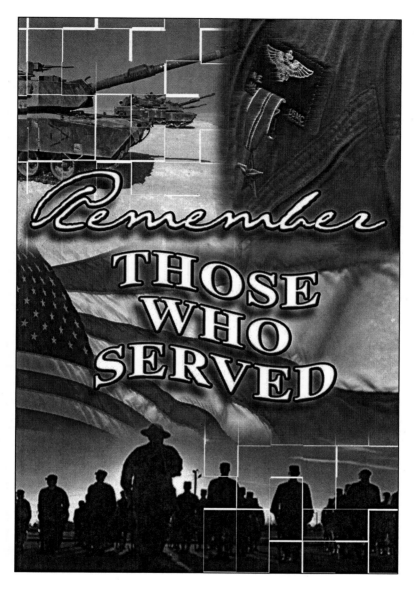

In Memory of Barney Humiston- story pg. 99
Designed by Nikki Griffin

3 End-of-Life Decisions

There are many decisions that we make throughout our lifetime, some impulsive and some well-thought out. How we choose to worship, the partners we have chosen, the children we have helped raise, the community we live in, and the physicians who have cared for us will all play an important role in our end-of-life decisions. These decisions may take on a new perspective as we contemplate what care we want provided for us at the end of our lives and to whom we entrust the management of our affairs or estate. The following guidelines are to inform you about issues or directives you may need to address and are not considered a substitute for legal counsel.

Patient's Bill of Rights

If you have ever been in a hospital, health care facility or doctor's office than more than likely you noticed the *Patient's Bill of Rights* posted on the wall. Certain rights and responsibilities must be followed to ensure the best of care is provided to all patients. Here are five very brief summations from the twelve *Bill of Rights* that are written by *The American Hospital Association*: 1. The right to privacy, 2. The right to an Advance Directive, 3. The right to make decisions about one's plan of care, 4. The right to know of charges for services rendered, and 5. The right to considerate and respectful care.

To review the complete *Patient's Bill of Rights* visit *The American Hospital Association* website at http://www.aha.org.

Advance Directives

Through the *Patient Self-Determination Act of 1990*, the Federal Law requires that patients be provided with information on *Advance Directives* upon admission to a health care facility. In order to ensure one's wishes are acknowledged regarding health care and treatments, whether at the end of life or during an incident of incapacity, these documents or *Directives* need to be completed while one is deemed capable. These documents must be appropriately witnessed then copies given to those who need to know, which may include family members, physicians, health facility, and your lawyer. Any of them can be revoked or amended at any time. The following is a brief synopsis of *Advance Directives*:

A *Living Will* designates one's desire to use or not use life prolonging care during a terminal or irreversible condition or vegetative state. Desired care can be specific in regard to mechanical ventilation/respiration, use of intravenous fluids or a feeding tube, symptom management, and/or use of aggressive therapy.

A *Health Care Power of Attorney or Surrogate/HCS* designates a person or persons to make medical decisions and provide consent for health care if one is deemed unable to make those decisions for themselves.

A *Durable Power of Attorney/DPOA* designates a person or persons to make decisions for one who is deemed unable to make decisions for themselves in relation to property, finances, living trust, legal matters, medical care, and other matters.

DNAR and *DNR* are acronyms for *Do Not Attempt Resuscitation* and *Do Not Resuscitate.* A terminally ill patient who does not wish efforts taken to be revived if their breathing or heart stops must sign this form, along with their physician. The person designated as the *Health Care Surrogate* or *Durable Power of Attorney* may sign on behalf of the patient if he/she is incapacitated.

Organ or Anatomical Donation is the transferring of certain organs, tissues, or cells from a deceased donor to a recipient. This individual request can be noted on a Driver's License or State Identification Card and be submitted to your state donor registry. If there is no designation of donor wishes but family members, HCS, or one's DPOA feel this may be something the deceased would have wanted to do, then those with proper authority can consent for donation. There is detailed information at http://organdonor.gov/donor/index.htm. We will discuss organ donation further in Chapter Four.

If you would like more information about *Advance Directives* and need it in a language other than English, you can access *Five Wishes* at http://www.agingwithdignity.org/ where you can order *Advance Directive* forms that are available in twenty languages. Please note that at this time not all states accept these forms as legal documents. Even if your state does not yet recognize *Five Wishes,* it still provides a wealth of information to you. To view sample documents specific to your State of residence, http://www.caringinfo.org/stateaddownload is the Internet site to review. Numerous websites address the same concerns and needs. Please *remember to use legal counsel to ensure proper legal documentation.*

Additional Documents or Directives

A *legal will* is a written document that ensures that after your death there is no misunderstanding as to whom you wish your estate or property to go to, who the guardian should be for any underage children, and who the executor or personal representative of the will is. A will can be self-compiled or completed with the assistance of a lawyer. Using legal counsel to ensure proper completion and wording is recommended. If there is no will written then the State court determines how the property is distributed and, if required, who will obtain custody of the children. Some States allow only partial distribution of property to one's spouse and children before the court decides on estate distribution and may even place limits on access to bank funds very soon after one's death. Unfortunately, the majority of Americans have not written a will so one's end of life wishes may not be fulfilled and court decisions may be further delayed. For more information on wills research http://www.aarp.org at the *American Association of Retired Persons* or phone 1-888-687-2277.

A perfect example in the importance of having a will occurred after the death of one of my hospice patients. This elderly lady needed someone to care for her during her last months of life so she asked her granddaughter to permanently move in with her. The grandmother *verbally* promised the granddaughter, who had several young children, that she would inherit her house after her death and so it was assumed that would occur. Very unfortunately, there was no will ever written to that effect. So upon an earlier than expected death of the grandmother, the granddaughter and her children came home after school and discovered the house locks changed, leaving them with no claim to any belongings inside.

Writing a will may seem like a premature thing to do in our younger years but it can be life impacting if not done, especially if an unexpected or earlier than expected death occurs.

Right to Die

Lois Gerber is a nurse who faced the same decisions and challenges as any adult child concerning their parent's end of life care. Her story addresses Advance Directives on a heart wrenching scale:

The ringing telephone jarred me awake in the middle of the night. "It's Andrea, your mother's nurse. I hate to have to call you like this, but your mother has had a heart attack. Can you come now?"

As a community health nurse, I realized what this new complication could mean. As a daughter, I was scared. I knew things weren't going well. Three days after my mother's surgery to remove a brain tumor, she was still on a ventilator unconscious in the neurological ICU. Earlier that night, I had left the hospital with an uneasy feeling. Once I got home and ate a late dinner, I went to bed and fell into a restless sleep.

I stumbled out of bed and dressed in the slacks and shirt I had just taken off. My mind was a blur as I got in my car and drove the ten miles to the hospital. I parked in the near-empty lot and raced to the elevator to ride to the ICU on the seventh floor.

The neurosurgeon, Doctor Reed, met me in the hallway. I sensed anxiety and compassion in his eyes. "Your mother is in heart failure," he told me. "She had a heart attack two hours ago. A cardiologist is with her now. Her blood gases have been poor. The heart complications have caused brain death."

I felt the blood drain from my face. "I can't believe this happened," I gasped.

"We all feel awful." He took my arm and led me through the swinging doors into the ICU.

Still in shock, I walked hesitantly to my mother's bed. She looked the same as she did when I left six hours earlier— the turban of white bandages wrapped around her head, clear liquid dripping into a vein in her arm through IV tubing, the monitor leads connected to her chest.

Yet I also saw evidence of her deteriorating condition. A chest X-ray, left at the bedside, showed her lungs were filled with fluid. And on closer inspection I noticed that her level of consciousness had decreased.

Doctor Reed pointed to the monitor. "Premature ventricular contractions characteristic of damaged heart muscle. We got the fluid out of her lungs but too late to reverse the brain damage. Because of the fresh brain surgery, we couldn't chance any clot dissolving or blood thinning medications."

I was suddenly aware of someone standing at my elbow. It was Andrea, my mom's nurse. Andrea first noticed the change in my mother's condition and instituted a code on her. Because of Andrea, Mom was still alive.

She squeezed my arm gently, and then focused her attention on Mom. I watched her add medicine to her IV and draw blood from an artery in her hand. She explained what she was doing. Mom lay there seemingly not able to hear. When she finished the procedures, she rubbed her hand across Mom's forehead. Her skill and gentleness soothed me. "What do you think?" I asked.

She guided me into a family conference room where there was a table and several chairs. I sat down and laid my head on the table. Andrea sat quietly. When I raised my head and asked, "What happened?" she squeezed my arm and handed me a tissue.

"We had a tough time stabilizing her. The heart and brain are severely affected." Her words reinforced what the neurosurgeon had already told me.

I knew I had some tough decisions to make. Being a nurse and only child wouldn't make them any easier. Andrea offered to help me sort through the options for Mom's care. We discussed the pros and cons of a full code, quality of life issues, and the hospital's *Dying Patient's Bill of Rights*, where a dying person has the right to have a family member or close friend sit with them. "Take your time making the decision," she said.

I remembered how Mom used to say, "Everyone dies when it is the right time. Let me go when my time comes."

I told Andrea that Mom didn't want to be kept alive with life support. Her medical directive paperwork confirmed this. I had already been appointed medical power of attorney and had no one I needed to consult. I decided to honor Mom's wishes and immediately stop the cardiac medications and only continue the comfort drugs. The physician concurred. "You're very brave," Andrea told me.

"Thank you for being here for us. I needed someone like you to understand how I felt and to listen to me."

"It's what we nurses do, isn't it?" she said.

Typically, in the ICU, family members can only visit with the patient for only short time periods every hour. Andrea interceded with her nurse manager so that I could sit at my mother's bedside continually throughout the night. She brought me coffee and massaged my shoulders.

Andrea's presence, the closeness of my mother's body, and the strangely reassuring drone of the ventilator and flashing monitors comforted me. I sat quietly crying into a pillow at the head of my mother's bed. Andrea pulled up a chair and sat with me for a few minutes every hour or so. At dawn, as the sun started to light the sky, my mother's heart stopped. She died peacefully as she would have wanted. The ventilator was turned off.

Andrea held me and cried with me. "This is the hard part of nursing made beautiful," she said.

I spent only eight hours with Andrea but felt an intimate connection to her. Her skill, empathy, and sensitivity turned a traumatic experience into a meaningful life lesson.

Being on the receiving end of nursing reminded me that we, as nurses and as people, can have a profound effect on others in times of crises. Andrea's caring and compassion gave me the support I needed to deal with my overwhelming grief, confusion, and vulnerability.

Hester's Last Smile

Whether the dying resides in a shelter, their own home, a health related facility, or a penthouse in an oceanside condominium makes no difference when it comes to making their final choices. Each should be provided the respect and dignity all humans deserve. Bob Ellenberg is present to support one special lady in her final decisions and hours of life:

Hester is in her mid fifties, dying of cancer. She was a street woman known at the local shelter where she came occasionally needing a meal or a place to stay. As a younger woman, she worked, had a marriage and children. Now she only has one eighteen-year-old daughter who has been visiting. I asked when she saw the other children. She tries to whisper something to me but can't get the words out because her tracheotomy is clogged with mucous. She puts up ten thin fingers, makes a fist and holds them up again.

"Twenty years?" She smiles and nods.

Hester has throat cancer, which has now metastasized throughout her abdomen, putting her in excruciating pain that is relieved by strong doses of medications ordered by her physician. None of it seems enough to deaden the pain. I am promised by the hospice nurse that Hester will soon be on the intravenous Morphine pump and she will be able to give herself as much as she can take.

This is Hester's second time in the nursing home where I work as a social worker. She came in carrying two large cans of cheap rolling tobacco, one tucked under each arm. As I pointed at her coming down the hall, I gave her a friendly, welcome laugh. She laughed back knowing she was a different kind of picture.

What am I to do for her? Get down on my hands and knees and pray that she doesn't have too much pain. Should I ask God to help her go fast or that she be miraculously healed? I know that's not what is up for her. She's on her way from this life. She told me she is ready to die, especially with all the pain. I don't want her to have the pain. I don't want her to suffer. I want her to have a chance but I'm not sure a chance at what.

I watched her sitting outside on the patio with the other smokers limply holding a long ashed cigarette in her emaciated fingers. Her breathing was gargled through her tracheotomy. I looked at her very wrinkled face, more of an eighty-year-old than someone in her fifties. I feel saddened by her circumstance.

Her few teeth are black and rotten. Still, her smile remains bright, frequent and I wonder if I will ever see it again. I've gotten attached to her.

The hospice social worker and I make arrangements with a local mortuary for her requested cremation. I asked Hester if she wants me to spread her remains on Paynes Prairie, the thousands of acres of natural, pristine Florida, with birds, alligators, giant turtles, herons, deer, transplanted buffalo, and wild horses. She nodded. I think about her soon turning to ash, which is more like gritty, rough sand.

A few days later she can barely sit up, barely take anything to drink, hasn't eaten much in the four weeks she has been with us, her eyes closed most of the time, occasional tremors, grimaces on her face, and no smiles except a very slight corner of the mouth smile when the hospice nurse got real close to her face and made a joke.

Hester's' eighteen-year-old daughter, Leola, is in the room with Hester. Leola signed the *Do Not Resuscitate* order at the behest of Hester.

The hospice nurse is explaining to Hester and Leola that if a feeding tube was put in, because of her condition, her body might react by the lungs collecting some of the liquid and she may aspirate. The surgery may be too much for her. Hester is more alert this morning then all week so she understands, shaking her head *no* about the feeding tube. For two days, Hester has been sitting up, enjoying the time with Leola and her two-year-old son.

I joke about her missing her own baptism while she was in a sleepy state. Hester wanted to be baptized so a Catholic priest performed the sacred ritual, answering all the questions himself that he asked of Hester. He explained to me this is the way it is done in these circumstances.

Hester's drinking only a bit of the nutritional supplements, a sip of water now and then. Each day she asks me, "When? How much longer?" I tell her, "You have to wait your turn; there are others ahead of you." I was surprised as she looked deeply into my eyes, nodding that she understood.

The eye connection we are having is leaving a deep and, I know forever, lasting impression on me. I can feel the imprinting going on. I have the realization that many I help like this, and for all of us whoever we are with, become us, we them, as our life is literally transformed from each and every experience we are having in this life and we're becoming all that has ever been.

I sat with Hester yesterday watching her twitch and wiggle around a bit. She looked pitifully weak and down with this life. Off and on she opened her eyes a crack and looked at me, but wasn't able nor was it necessary for her to acknowledge my presence. I patted her hand, rested my hand on her forehead for a few moments, brushed back her hair with my fingers, and whispered to her that it wasn't going to be much longer. There was no response except when I asked her if she wanted a blanket or sheet and she mouthed *sheet*. As I covered her I wished her the best, hoping she didn't have to continue the ordeal much longer.

When I came to work the next morning, the mortician was wheeling her past my office. Just in time to say one last good-bye.

Dorothy's Story

Hospice Nurse Barbara Richford reflects on a death with dignity when a prolonged life is allowed to end:

Dorothy was the matriarch of the nursing home where she lived. When she arrived seven years ago she won the hearts and minds of the entire staff through her pleasantness and generosity. Her love of dancing and partying touched their spirit. When she became restless and began wandering they busied her with folding laundry and she would be content. When she was tired she would sit in her beautiful room overlooking the pond on the grounds where her grandchildren attended school. She would munch on cookies and offer some to anyone who entered her room.

The time came when Dorothy needed to move on but the staff could not let her go and convinced the family to prolong her life, promising that the quality of her life would improve. Instead, Dorothy retreated more and more into herself while her body declined into a frozen state. The family grieved the decision they were compelled to make and thought they could not change it.

Then one day a hospice program was implemented and Dorothy became a candidate for it. The family accepted this with great enthusiasm, as finally Dorothy would receive what she needed. The day the feeding tube was stopped was a day to remember. The Head Nurse herself stopped the feeding and everyone gathered around Dorothy to say good-bye, cry and reminisce. It was there that I learned of Dorothy's history.

Dorothy slipped away just as she lived. Her vital signs never changed nor did her breathing pattern, which is unusual for a dying person. She lasted a long time given her age and condition. However, as I reflect on her uniqueness, this is consistent of how she lived and conducted her life. She did it her way with dignity, grace and beauty.

I went to Dorothy's wake and was astounded by her complete rejuvenation and transformation. The family left the casket open after seeing how she looked. Although she was ninety-eight when she died, she did not look a day older than seventy in her comfortable coffin, in her beautiful outfit, surrounded by flowers and a loving, devoted family.

I learned from Dorothy's case that staff can hold onto us because of their influence on the family, believing it's not time to die. Not recognizing that life does end causes most of the problems we are seeing in the traditional medical setting today. This view takes on an unspoken rule that we as a human race defy the way things are. The scientific model does not explore the spiritual or human side of life and death therefore it has nothing built into it to cope with failure. The separation of beginnings and endings causes great pain and struggle for those who just need to move on. Because death is equated with failure, everything may be done to continue to sustain life without regard to quality of life. The person who needs to die may suffer much more than is necessary.

Dorothy is free now and her death freed those around her. Eventually the problems of incorrect thinking will change when enough people do enough suffering to wake other people up to a possibility of thinking differently. Farewell, dear Dorothy, and thank you for your life and contribution to making the human race better than the way you found it.

Avoiding Anxiety

End-of-life concerns and legal decisions are something each of us should resolve during our healthier days. But unfortunately many are deferred until one is close to death and/or incapacitated. With a timely *open awareness,* the anxiety involved with such critical and complex issues can be significantly reduced through discussion and education. That is my wish for you.

4 Just Past the Final Hour

The phone book was opened to the yellow pages as the headlines of *Funeral Directors* and *Funeral Planning* boldly lay before Jane's eyes. The yellow was turning to blotches of gray as her tears slowly toppled from her cheeks. Her trembling finger glided over the headlines as she kept repeating, "Why now? Why now? Why now?"

Instead of Jane being able to spend all of her last precious moments at her loved one's bedside, she was faced with perhaps hasty decisions in how to best pay tribute to her husband. Her decisions, that would reflect their beliefs, values, and familial customs, would be remembered and replayed in her mind for years to come.

If pre-planning for one's final care has not been done then numerous life impacting decisions must be made in just a matter of hours. Those decisions can include what type of service will be held and where will it be, in the funeral home, your church or possibly your own home, what should be included in one's obituary, should you choose cremation or burial, which casket or urn do you desire, where should you bury your loved one or spread their ashes, and what will the expenses be.

Jane quickly realized the transition through these end-of-life hours would have been less distressing if only her and her husband had discussed these issues days, months, or even years prior to his death. With pre-planning, Jane and her husband would have been able to visit several funeral homes and decide which one could best fulfill both their needs.

It is too late to offer some guidance to Jane but it is not for you, so let us get started and get some answers to many questions my hospice families and end-of-life students ask about funeral services.

The Funeral Rule and The General Price List

A benefit to Jane and anyone else faced with funeral decisions is a law that has been in effect since 1984 by *The United States Federal Trade Commission* called *The Funeral Rule*. Because significant sums of money for after death care may incur, part of this rule mandates that all funeral providers must offer the bereaved or other clients an accurate and written *General Price List* before final choices have been made. This list includes such things as charges for professional services of the Funeral Director and staff that are non-declinable, embalming and cremation costs, casket prices (you are allowed to buy a casket from an outside source, have a talented woodworker make one for you, or may be able to rent a casket for the service), an outer burial container if required by a cemetery, death certificates, use of funeral facilities, equipment and/or vehicles, graveside services, and forwarding or receiving the deceased from another funeral home. Purchases for single items can be made and/or a package may be available, which might include numerous ancillary items such as a photo collage, memorial folders, flowers, prayer cards, memorial candle, etc.

Most funeral homes have chapels that are available for wakes, funerals, or memorial services. Typically, crematoriums do not have chapels. If desired, one's own church can be used for services instead of a funeral home and would typically have a lower expense involved. Many hospice facilities have their own chapel where hospice patients and families may choose to hold their service.

A celebration of one's life can include some very moving tributes and include some very unique items. One gentleman wanted his motorcycle at his memorial service so it was positioned in the front of the chapel while his riding partners recalled fond memories of their travels together.

Something that was common years ago, and is more common in other countries, is holding the wake and service in one's home. That is my father's request and our family will do our best to honor his wishes in our hometown in northern New York.

A question that is occasionally asked is how much should it cost to have one's remains transported a short or long distance from their town of residence to their chosen resting place? It is common for a funeral provider to have a transport cost considered as part of their basic service, usually within a twenty-five to fifty-mile radius. On the *General Price List* from a funeral provider, an accurate charge for transporting must be listed. If a longer distance is required the local funeral provider can assist you in arranging transport, whether by plane or van, and inform you of the cost involved. Your local funeral home and the out-of-area funeral home remain in close communication so timely arrangements can be made with the proper paperwork and permits obtained. If pre-planning has been done then, upon the death of your loved one, the first phone call should be to the funeral home where your pre-planning was done. More expenses may incur with the use of a second funeral home so be sure to clarify that with your funeral provider.

A widow wished to have her loved one buried twelve hundred miles away where they had purchased two cemetery spaces years prior. She had a limited income and could not afford the extra cost of $950 to have him transported by plane. So after her husband was embalmed, placed in a casket, then placed in her mini-van, their son drove north to their hometown funeral home with the proper paperwork and permits in hand.

Pre-planning and Pre-paying

There are individuals who are in favor of pre-paying for funeral services and those who prefer not to. Pre-planning is definitely advantageous, as Jane discovered, and it can be done with or without paying anything at the time of decision-making. The advantage of pre-paying offers less concern because you offset an increase in costs by locking-in the price. However, that leads to my next question.

What happens if your pre-paid funeral provider closes his or her business or changes ownership? When a licensed Funeral Home is to be sold, the State Regulatory Agency must approve the sale and requires by law that pre-paid monies must stay the same and must be honored. Remember that your questions or concerns are *free-to-ask* of your funeral provider by phone or in person.

Expenses for funeral services can vary significantly, even between funeral homes within just a few miles of each other. Just like any other important decision, it pays to compare facilities, staff, and costs. In my hometown, the *average* cost for cremation ranges from $800 to $1,000 and the *average* cost for a funeral service with embalming can range from $5,000 to $6,500. Certainly expenditures can vary depending on the services and items chosen, with even tens of thousands of dollars more being added to the cost.

Finding Funds

For those concerned about acquiring funds to pay for funeral services or medical expenses there are several options but you must carefully research each. If you have a life insurance policy, you may be qualified for a *Viatical Settlement* or an *Accelerated Death Benefit/ADB* that allows terminal patients to obtain a portion of their policy funds prior to their death. One must use great caution in who they consult before deciding on a settlement because, unfortunately, honesty is not everyone's policy. Also, Funeral Homes will take an Insurance Policy Assignment. For more information you can contact your Funeral Director, your trusted insurance agent, or research information at *The National Association of Insurance Commissioners* at http://www.naic.org/, which offers many articles relating to these topics. It is always wise to use legal counsel.

Another option in acquiring funds is through a *Reverse Mortgage*, which provides senior homeowners cash based on the equity of their home. Some close friends of mine obtained a *Reverse Mortgage* through *The United States Department of Housing and Urban Development, which is* known as *HUD,* and they are very pleased with their decision. Research http://www.hud.gov/buying/rvrsmort.cfm or call 1-(202) 708-1112 for more information.

Embalming

The practice of preserving bodies by embalming is thought to have begun with the Egyptians, prior to 4000BC. Through the use of numerous substances, such as herbs, salts, spices, aloes and wax, many have been preserved for hundreds of years in vaults. Eventually the practice of embalming spread to Europe then on to America where its use increased during the Civil War in an effort to preserve the fallen soldier who was a distance from his home.

Today, embalming pertains to the removal of body fluids and replacing it with a preservative solution. A greater expense is involved with embalming over cremation because it entails much more. Approximately sixty percent of those embalmed are also cremated.

Embalming does not provide a permanent preservation but rather delays decomposition. It may be required by a Funeral Home for a public visitation.

Cremation

Cremation, the reduction of one's body to ashes through the use of heat, has been traced back to about 3000BC. It was introduced to the western world by the Greeks around 1000BC when fallen soldiers were cremated and their ashes returned to their homeland. Cremation was also done for safety and health reasons when dangerous plagues killed thousands of people in the mid-1600s.

The first crematorium in the United States was opened in 1876. Not all funeral homes have their own crematoriums so they contract one in their area.

Nearly all religions approve of cremation, with the exceptions of Eastern Orthodox, Orthodox Jews, Islamic and several Fundamentalist Christians.

Direct cremation is typically requested when no visitation or viewing is desired at the funeral or memorial service. A simpler casket made of cardboard is most often used for cremation. The ashes or cremains have the consistency of a coarse powder or coral, which are placed in a container of the loved one's choosing, called an urn.

When a service is held after the cremation, the ashes are often placed in an urn, which is positioned among cherished photos, keepsakes, and special memorabilia that represents the life of one so loved. Loved one's ashes may be spread *usually* where the family chooses, whether on land, at sea, or from the air, but if burial is chosen then purchasing a space or mausoleum will be an added expense.

State Laws mandate a waiting period prior to a cremation taking place. In the State of Florida, a forty-eight hour waiting period is required. Your local Funeral Director will inform you of the laws and answer any questions you may have about cremation. *The Internet Cremation Society* offers more information and includes pictures taken inside a crematorium at http://www.cremation.org/.

Ashes and Joy

A hospice nurse and co-worker of mine named Mary Freeman shares a great story related to ashes that will cause you to chuckle. Bring on the joy, Mary!

One day my grandchildren, Little Charlie, Tommy, and Daisy, were playing inside my son Charlie's house. They were running their cars and trucks through a dirt road, making tracks along the way.

Because my son didn't appreciate them bringing dirt inside, he yelled at them for doing just that.

Then Little Charlie explained that he didn't bring in the dirt but got it from a bag in the closet. His dad soon realized it was his beloved Grandma's ashes.

Charlie's wife, Dawn, took it very well because she said that Grandmother loved little kids and considered them to be a great blessing.

So they swept up the rest of the ashes and scattered them around outside where Grandma would want to be. Now don't you think Grandma had a hand in that?

The Pets We Have Loved

Many of us have taken our young children to the back of our lawns to bury our precious pets and hold a memorial service. These events provide us with *teachable moments* that begin the process of understanding that death comes to us all.

Our pets provide us unconditional love and so it is very understandable that we grieve over their death. It is important to provide closure whether through a simple backyard burial, to purchasing or making a specialty marker, or providing an urn for their ashes. Funeral providers and specialty pet shops offer an array of items for our pets, with many items also available on-line.

My brother Bruce says that if his dog Rocky isn't in heaven than he doesn't want to go there. Well, I most definitely believe Rocky is there and also our family dog, Spooky. Countless others, from priests to pastors to prophets, believe the same.

Caskets and Urns

When it comes to cost, the casket is usually the top of the price list for consumers whether purchased at the funeral home or at a casket store. An approximate low-end price for a casket is $1,000, with much pricier caskets ranging beyond $7,000. A plain pine casket can be purchased for approximately $600. Most caskets are made of steel, wood, or fiberglass, with or without a seal.

Urns can be purchased for approximately $30 but also have a wide variance in price. There are many different styles of keepsake urns and many beautiful pieces of jewelry that are designed to hold a tiny portion of ashes. A dove necklace of Barbara Graham's holds her mother's ashes, pictured on page 73.

The funeral home must honor whatever casket or urn you choose when obtained from another source, whether purchased online or in-store. You may be able to rent a casket for the service and then use a less expensive one for burial or cremation. It may be financially worthwhile to inquire at several funeral homes about the types of casket rentals. A funeral home charge for a casket rental averages $500-$1200.

If there is a woodworker in the family, a casket kit or directions can be purchased and then a casket fabricated with very loving hands. Instructions are easy to find on the Internet or ask for assistance in your local bookstore or library.

Traditional Cemetery

A ground burial in a traditional cemetery has its own related fees that are separate from funeral provider costs, which may include a cemetery space and possibly an outer burial container. An outer burial container is a concrete container in which the casket is lowered. Its purpose is to maintain level ground and support the use of heavy maintenance equipment without harming the caskets. There are no mandated laws that say an outer burial container must be used but cemeteries can require it. An average price of an outer burial container is $700-$1200.

A cemetery space can be purchased for a single burial or for multiple burials that will provide space for other family members. Depending on where the space is depends on the cost. I found numerous cemetery spaces for sale on the Internet with the minimal single space price at $1500 then upward to $5,000.

It is important to ask cemetery owners about opening and closing fees, vault and headstone setting fees, ground keeping and perpetual upkeep fees. Some of these fees may be included in the space purchase but one should not assume so.

When a casket or urn is to be entombed in a mausoleum crypt, niche, or columbarium, (which are buildings typically above ground), various costs and fees also apply.

Green Burial in a Green Cemetery

Green Burial sites allow for the deceased to return to nature through a natural decaying process at a much cheaper cost than a traditional burial. Usually, the wake and the funeral are held in the home. The deceased is placed in a biodegradable product that decomposes over time. There are numerous locations of *Green Cemeteries* and each must observe all state regulations and health requirements. For more information about Green Burials visit the *Green Burial Council* site at http://www.greenburialcouncil.org/.

Writing the Obituary, Completing Forms

Upon meeting with your Funeral Director, he or she will assist you in compiling the information for your loved one's newspaper notice or obituary. Information you may want to provide may include your loved one's parents' names, immediate family members and survivors, schools attended, occupational background, suggested memorial donations, personal accomplishments, and funeral or memorial service information. There may be an extra charge by the newspaper for obituaries and the inclusion of a picture.

For required forms and paperwork, your Funeral Director will ask you to provide your loved one's birth date, Social Security number, and Veteran's Discharge Papers.

The Department of Veterans Affairs Benefits

After reading the next story you will know why it is very important to me that the *United States of America* honors those who have died while serving their country. For detailed information about veterans' funeral and memorial benefits visit the *Department of Veterans Affairs* website at http://www.cem.va.gov/ or phone 1-800-827-1000. Another Internet website you may find to be helpful is at http://www.military.com/benefits/burial-and-memorial. In Chapter Five, you will learn about *TAPS*, which offers tremendous support for our Armed Forces surviving family members, who we should never forget nor the sacrifices they also made.

The *Arlington National Cemetery* in Washington D.C. is well known for its availability to those who have served in the Armed Forces. There are also many other National cemeteries throughout our country where veterans can be buried. Free Veteran benefits include a cemetery space and one also for his/her spouse, an outer burial container, a memorial stone, and the Professional Service Fee. Active duty military honors are available to all Veterans. Your funeral home provider will have further veteran information.

Dying for their Country

The memory of my Uncle Barnum Humiston, who was killed in the Korean War, is carried with me in every visit I make with my veteran patients. Certainly no one would have expected the news of his death in September of 1952 to be delivered in such an unfathomable manner. My Aunt Donnamae tells the heartrending story about her only brother, my Uncle Barney:

Although it has been fifty-five years ago, it seems like yesterday from the pain I have in my heart. It is very hard for me to talk about it as tears come to my eyes.

It was a sunny, warm day in September. We had not heard from Barney for about two weeks. He had been in the service for such a short time, around six months, so it was surprising that he was sent to Korea so soon. Troops were needed and although it was not called a war there was much fighting and many lives lost. Barney was an only son and could have chosen not to go to Korea but he wanted to go and get it over with.

My brother liked music and could play any instrument as it came to him very easy- guitar, banjo, violin, plus chords on the piano. He did all jobs on the farm and started driving tractor when he was very young. He liked cars and knew every make and model. He would go down to Bangor and visit Uncle Frank at the gas station and help him. Sometimes he would meet some friends there, of which he had many.

Before he left for Korea, Barney had just a few days at home in June. He told me that if he did not return to take good care of Mom and Dad. I think he had a feeling he would not be coming back.

While in the Army, Barney was a sharp shooter and drove a big tank. He was in the tank Battalion as a Private. Barney had one close friend in the Army but he went to Paris when Barney went to Korea.

During this time, Dad was working for a neighbor farmer and I was in grade school, which had already started. Shirley, my sister, was married to Carlton and was pregnant with their third child.

The morning we found out, I was sleeping in an upstairs bedroom. Mom woke me up to get ready for school. It was early. Dad had already left for work after milking our three or four cows.

Once downstairs, she opened one of the front doors, which we never used, because it was a very warm day and she wanted to let in some air.

I came down stairs and Mom said she had found a telegram inside the front door. As she read it, she said Barney had been wounded, and then she said, "Oh no! Barney has died...he was killed in action!"

We do not know how long the message had been there. The message could have been there for days. He died September 5. I turned thirteen on September 6.

Barney's body came by train and was escorted by one soldier. That was his job in the service to be with the family and with the deceased until the burial. They arrived in North Bangor, New York and Barney was picked up by Spaulding's Funeral Home, which was in Bangor at that time.

The wake was at the funeral home and the service was at the Methodist Church in Bangor. School was let out for the funeral and there were so many at the church that there was not enough room so some were outside. There was a large crowd at the cemetery with military rites and a 21-gun salute with the bugle that plays.

Barney was buried December 10th, on his birthday. He would have been twenty-two.

My Uncle Barney, who I never got to meet, would want you to remember that nearly 37,000 servicemen and women died in the Korean War, nearly 100,000 were wounded, and over 8,000 are listed as missing in action.

It would be grand if a veteran that knew Barney would contact me, as noted on the copyright page, so I could share your words with Barney's only siblings, my Aunt Donnamae and my mother Shirley. A big thank you goes out to all of you who have served and suffered for our country so the rest of us can live in a land of the free.

Joy in Artifacts

There are many precious items that come to mind when we think of those who cherished them and held them close: the American flag, Medals of Honor, jewelry, special collectibles, dolls, teddy bears, love letters, clothing, etc. Such items have strong memories attached to them and can be placed with the deceased temporarily or permanently, whether in the casket or during cremation. These precious items are known as *funerary artifacts*.

Many tender memories come to mind of loved ones who have placed copies of precious photos inside a pocket, laid a favorite lap robe across their Mom's body, placed a golf tee inside a buddy's shirt pocket, tucked a keepsake doll under Grandma's arm, pinned a medal on a veteran's collar, put a favored locket around Auntie's neck, and laid a military dogtag by a father's side. Our next story, told by Marion Staples, is about some very special *funerary artifacts* passed from a son to his father:

It was the end of February 2007 when I received a call from my sister that her husband, Anthony, had lost his long battle with lung cancer. I flew to Connecticut to be with my family and attend the service. This was the family that opened their arms to me after my husband passed away nine years ago. I would spend Christmas holidays with them and a few weeks during the summer.

The wake, the funeral, and the reception were all scheduled on the same day. The weather was not very pleasant as it was cold, windy, rainy and sometimes snowing. The immediate family gathered at the funeral home for some private time before the wake started for the rest of the visitors.

My sister and her husband had just one child, Anthony, Jr. When he and his wife and their three daughters arrived, they approached the coffin. While saying their final good-byes and offering prayers, we watched as his son pinned two "very special" fishing flies on the lapel of his father's suit jacket. This was a very touching moment, a remembrance of the many times they had gone fly fishing together.

His father's passion for his last twenty-five years was tying all of his own flies and these "very special flies" that his son refers to as "crazy Brown and White Bivisible" is what he would use when nothing else would work. This fly did not look like anything special and from the purist point of view should never cause a trout to look at it. But his Dad could catch fish on this fly when no one else even got a strike!!! It was all "catch and release" except for two special catches that he had mounted.

Following the wake, we moved on to the church for the 2:00pm Mass, followed by Military Honors performed on the church steps, still in the wind, rain and snow. I think the taps were played while the player sat in a car in the parking lot with the car window open!

During the Mass, scriptures were read by the granddaughters, followed by a wonderful and moving eulogy given by his son, Anthony.

The first part of his eulogy covered the very full life of the eighty years of this very talented, diverse, extraordinary man who strived for perfection in all of his endeavors, his life-long career building and remodeling homes, filling his leisure time with golf, bowling, skiing, motorcycling, fly fishing, being an avid Yankee fan and UCONN basketball fan, attending most all of his son's sporting events when he was growing up and most of his granddaughter's sporting events- a very full life.

Anthony finished the eulogy by sharing his last fishing experience with his father while sitting by his bedside in the hospital. They were at the Farmington River, a fish was rising under a branch, a spot in the Park where Dad had previoiusly caught a few two and three pound fish. I thought it was a brown, not Dad, he clearly uttered "rainbow." I said we should try a "nymph". He clearly said "ant."

It was quiet for a few minutes while Dad was thinking then his right hand shook and he uttered, "I've got a big one!!"

I asked, "How big?"

A couple of minutes went by then he said, "15!"

"Is that inches or pounds?"

He quickly answered, "I don't know'"

He rested quietly for a few more minutes. I asked if he needed me to net the fish.

"NO!!", he exclaimed.

That was Dad, stubborn to the end.

May God bless him and show him the best trout streams heaven has to offer. I am so happy I had a chance to share that fishing trip with him in heaven.

A Memory Jar

Do you have treasured memorabilia from your loved one who has passed that may include old buttons, a broken locket, special coins, pieces of jewelry, a marble, or dice, a tiny dollhead or stone? Years ago these treasures would be embedded in a putty-like substance on a vase or jar to hold precious tangible memories. Today you may find one of these beautiful jars displayed inside the walls of an antique store or in your family's attic.

One of my treasured friends has a wooden box that she keeps her husband's memorabilia in and when she sees something that reflects their bond of love, like a special card, she will buy it and tuck it inside her memory box.

If you have a special jar or box, maybe you would like to have it available at your loved one's service and request those attending to write down a special memory and tuck it inside for you to read later, during your own private time. It will be a precious way to begin your grieving process.

Markers and Headstones

There is a beautiful woman posed in prayer at a cemetery headstone in Manitowoc, Wisconsin, not far from where my husband Paul's parents are buried. I do not know the one who sculpted her or how long she has posed there but her stone body shows many years of aging. There are no words to describe the emotion in her posture and face so I have pictured her fully on page 72 and a portion of her on the cover.

In your town or in your travels be sure to glance into the cemeteries you pass as there are many gorgeous and unique headstones and monuments, also known as gravestones or tombstones, paying tribute to those who lie below. There is a pet cemetery north of Ocala, Florida that has a gorgeous statue of animals that I would like to share with you. It is pictured on page 74. Personally, I consider the choice of a gravestone or urn, which will be viewed for perhaps centuries to come, to hold a greater significance for survivors than the casket lying beneath the stone that was viewed for a handful of hours.

It is time to address another concern of my families and that is the expense of a gravestone, marker, monument or memorial bench and also pet markers. These items can range from a low cost of $150 to very elaborate gravestones of

$100,000. Be sure to ask if there are any additional cemetery costs or fees above the purchase of your marker.

After discovering that a cemetery space and casket alone may cost $6,000, it is easy to see why an average price for a funeral can quickly escalate to $10,000. (Many weddings don't even cost that much.) So why do some accumulate such expenses as they try to do their best in paying tribute to their loved one? I tend to believe we are emotionally weak and frail during our most intense hours of grief, and almost certainly in shock, so we may be less able to make the best of financial decisions. Obviously, when we are in our best of health is when we should pre-plan by making our funeral wishes known and pre-pay by locking in the price, allowing for payments to be made over time or paying the total sum. Either way, the burden of making funeral decisions is alleviated.

Wealth of Information

For those who desire more information about funeral planning and compliance, there is a wealth of information by *The Federal Trade Commission* at www.ftc.gov. Also, at http://www.funeralplan.com/ and http://www.funerals.org there are answers to questions you would never think to ask or think to be concerned about. Your local funeral home also offers compassionate care and guidance and can address many of your concerns. Education is empowering so learn all you can while you can. It just may save you some money and additional heartache.

Choose Wisely

Have you ever regretted not visiting someone who was dying or attending someone's funeral or memorial service? I have my regrets and it is not an easy thing to live with. So choose your funerals wisely. You will be thankful you did as your grief and your joy in knowing and remembering someone so loved will be shared with those who feel the same and are, like you, in their beginning stages of grieving.

Organ Donation

One of the most solemn of moments in my nursing career occurred while I was working in the Operating Room during an organ transplant. You could hear a pin drop. The surgery was performed with a reverence I had never experienced before.

Discussing organ donation is a very difficult and emotional topic to address. There are sixteen deaths a day due to a lack of organ donations as reported by The *Agency for Health Care Administration.* Major organs such as heart, liver, lungs, pancreas, intestines and kidneys can be donated, as well as blood vessels, heart valves, tissue, skin, eye corneas, and bone. It is likely that each of us already knows someone who was a donor and one who is a recipient. I met a woman who was given new corneas by grieving parents whose young child had died. Her gratitude and joy in being able to see her only children through the gift of another child was indescribable. She would like those parents to know how very grateful she is, as she has not met the mom and dad who so selflessly gave of their precious one.

There are no absolute age limits in being an organ donor but you must be 18 years of age to decide for yourself. Certain diseases such as an actively spreading cancer, severe and current infections, or a diagnosis of HIV will rule out a potential donor. The cost involved for the donor's organ transplantation is the responsibility of the recipient receiving the organ or tissue.

There are very strict guidelines that must be followed to allow for any transplant to occur. A team of medical professionals must determine the absence of vital signs without life sustaining equipment, plus the absence of brain or brain stem activity. The coordination involved between transplant agencies, medical professionals, and numerous support staff along with the timeliness of it all is paramount to a successful transplant.

Living donors have become more prevalent. When we talk about organ donation, it is common to hear discussions about a mother donating a kidney to her daughter, a lobe of a lung donated to a brother, or a portion of a pancreas donated to a diabetic child or adult. It is almost mind-boggling that our bodies have the power to heal others, as well as ourselves, yet we still must acknowledge the fact that we cannot live forever.

So you have the potential to improve the life of a very ill person who has little children to raise, a daughter who needs a new femur so she can walk down the aisle, a teacher who wants to visualize her students again, or a teenager whose heart won't allow him or her to play basketball or soccer.

Ok, now is the time to have an honest discussion with your family and loved ones and tell them how you feel. Gather as much information as you can, starting at your Driver's License Office, the *Transplant Living* website, or at the *US Organ Donor site at* http://www.organdonor.gov/. What a huge act of kindness and a legacy for you to leave behind as an organ donor.

Autopsy

There is no way we can address all the things we have without briefly discussing autopsy, which is a very detailed exam of the deceased by a Medical Examiner who is a physician. Autopsies are done for various reasons: if the death is suspicious, to help solve a crime, for identifying genetic or infectious diseases, if the death is an accident, as part of a teaching hospital's curriculum to train physicians, or if the death occurred at home without an attending physician to substantiate the death. Once the autopsy is done, the funeral provider cares for the deceased as the family desires.

Around the World

One of the things I most appreciated while working in Operating Rooms across this country was that my patients were all dressed alike in their *gorgeous* hospital acquired gown, no jewelry adorned them, and a paper bonnet covered their hair. It allowed for each of my patients to be presented in a near identical way without any notion of financial or hierarchical status, and without potential for prejudice.

My hospice patients certainly have different needs than those I cared for in the Operating Room. Yet it is still without prejudice that I attend to the dying, their families, and their loved ones, respecting their beliefs, customs, and values specific to their culture or family upbringing.

Even though there is a wide variety of funeral and burial rituals around the world, each of them has a very similar goal and that is to show great respect and honor for the dying and deceased. It is impossible in this text to state the uniqueness of each culture because many have adapted portions of other cultures due to mobilizing from one area to another. I would like to share some diversity of cultures of those who live within a short distance of each other in Central Florida and with whom I got to visit as a hospice nurse:

-at the bedside of an elderly gentleman who had just passed there was much emotion by his adult children with crying and pulling at one's clothes

-while visiting in a nursing home, it was very peaceful and quiet as the extended family sat in prayer at the bedside of their dying father, each reading scripture from the Bible

-two daughters in a small country home bathed and dressed their mother who had just passed, combed her hair then applied lipstick and rouge

-in a condominium no one was allowed to touch or see the deceased after his death

-one evening three young children were lying in bed next to their great-grandmother as she took her last breath

-two grandchildren were taken to the neighbor's house during the last hour before death and the deceased was removed before the children returned

In every home I enter, it is imperative that I do not instill my beliefs upon anyone but honor and respect the beliefs of the deceased and their loved ones, their choice of funeral services and body disposition, and their way of mourning. Universal compassion is paramount.

E-O-L Publishing Corporation would like to extend a sincere thank you to Nancy Lohman from *Lohman Funeral Homes*, Ormond Beach, Florida, for her input in this chapter.
www.lohmanfuneralhomes.com

5 Coping with Grief

Lying on the hospital bed with her face buried in her grandmother's pillow was Laura, the oldest of Mrs. M's six grandchildren. Her anticipatory grief was now realized as the reality and the shock surrounding her grandmother's death became evident. As Grandma M's body was removed from her home of eighty-seven years, sobs of loneliness spewed forth from Laura's throat. To her, the emotional pain of her grandmother's death was greater now than any physical pain she had ever endured.

Within the walls of this old country farmhouse was where Laura had spent countless, treasured hours tagging behind her grandmother, making cookies, casseroles, and anything else they could conjure up for their family, neighbors, and those less fortunate. All that Grandma M had taught Laura, kindness, gentleness, meekness, reverence, devotion, and compassion, along with the power of amazing grace, would remain with Laura forever. It was *filial piety*, a Chinese ideology, which her grandmother taught her for thirty-plus years. Grandmother M had learned the same from her parents, which included the importance of honoring one's parents and caring for them until their deaths. In those final hours, Laura promised her grandmother that her legacy would live on through her oldest grandchild and for generations to come.

But for now, Laura will cherish the warmth still present on her grandmother's bed and the sweet smell of her perfume deep-seated within the down of her pillow.

Anticipatory Grief

Perhaps over a time frame of weeks, months or even years, the very ill and their caregivers have anticipated certain events to occur as decline and death approach. This anticipatory grief or expected reaction to a loss may begin when *little deaths* occur such as being unable to fulfill employment, an increased dependence on others for personal care, needing to use a cane or walker, becoming wheelchair dependent or bed bound.

Those who have time to plan for an anticipated death tend to have a much greater acceptance of it, recognizing the need of what must be done, the decisions to be made and the time to make them. Stress may be diminished with a mutual awareness in knowing death is approaching.

Grief, Mourning, Bereaved

The way we react or respond physically, spiritually and emotionally to a death is termed grief. It is normal to exhibit certain signs and symptoms while in the process of grieving yet each is uniquely our own and transpires at our own pace. Mourning describes how we deal or cope with our grief, as we are confronted with our everyday responsibilities without our loved one present.

Those who are grieving and mourning after experiencing a recent death are often referred to as the bereaved. The ones I have attended to commonly exhibited two main behaviors. The first was a range of emotional responses where they often stayed very close to the bedside of the deceased as they cried tears of great sorrow, tears of joy in knowing and caring for one so loved, and/or tears of gratitude that the disease will no longer inflict harm on their loved one. Secondly, the survivor's behavior involved a more physical response with an active participation at the bedside with assisting in the final preparation of the deceased, tidying the room or home, and/or contacting those close to the family and friends. A blend of both behaviors seem to be the most common and the most comforting as mourning begins.

As the hours and days of loneliness evolve, grief may be exhibited physically in various ways such as with shortness of breath, lack of sleep, sensing emptiness in the pit of one's stomach, shaking as if chilled, a change in appetite and/or tightness in the chest or throat. As the griever yearns for the deceased, he or she may be on a constant watch in attempt to see them or find them in a crowd, hoping somehow the death cannot possibly be true.

Psychologically, the survivor is forced to cope without the loved one present and may require fulfilling duties that are unfamiliar. The increased stress of adapting alone may even cause depression, despair, or a weakened immune system.

Guilt can be a significant burden especially if the death was sudden or if the caregiver believes it is caused by their lack of care or attention to details. One's behaviors may change by isolating oneself from social events generally involved in, wanting to talk unceasingly about the deceased, directing feelings of anger on others, and having waves of strong emotions.

Many grievers will look for comfort in their church or religious community. If one believes the deceased's spirit is present then that may help sustain them as they adapt and learn how to adjust without their loved one's physical presence.

Other grievers may blame God for their loved one's death. Followers may even move away from their religion, perhaps returning to it once the heaviest weight of grief has eased and a purpose or meaning in the death has been established.

Comfort and Hope

One of Donnette R. Alfelt's books, titled *Comfort and Hope,* holds some very reassuring and encouraging words for widows, widowers and any others who are grieving. Donnette, a widow herself, explains how the grief process may evolve:

It is the nature of grief to be unpredictable and undulating. If you expect a steady climbing recovery you will be disappointed and discouraged. It is normal for life to be abnormal for a time. I recall times of peace when I felt at last I had made it through. I also remember these states being followed by relapses seemingly from nowhere or triggered by some small incident. There are uses served by the grief process, even in the tears. Tears of grief have ingredients that differ from tears of joy or laughter. This indicates that they have a special useful purpose that should not be denied. The phrase "a good cry" is understood by anyone who has had one. As much as we sometimes resist or even fight them, there is a change in us physically and emotionally after we let go and let the tears come.

Why I do What I do

I wish Donnette's book had been placed in my hands thirty years ago when I was first confronted with a loved one's death. My Grandpa Raymond died very suddenly in his northern New York home when his abdominal aortic aneurysm ruptured. Because I was very pregnant with my firstborn son, I was unable to travel the great distance to his funeral. I had a difficult time dealing with my grief partially because I didn't acknowledge it. I thought I was strong emotionally because I was a nurse and *knew* about death

Many years later when my best friend died suddenly of a heart attack at age fifty, grief again struck me with full force. I was devastated! Our sons were not only best buddies but she was my shopping partner, confidant and co-worker. We sat side by side on the bench at every ballgame our sons played together. We would shop for nearly nothing until we would drop. We solved all our problems together and created some we didn't know we had.

Several days after her heart attack, I was told she was in a comatose state and may not recover. I also learned that my friend had a vision of Heaven before she died. That was very comforting news and the first time I really became aware of near-death awareness.

With my anticipatory grief tucked way inside, I got up enough courage and held back my tears long enough to *visit* her in the intensive care unit. The nurse was hesitant to let me in because I wasn't family. (Who ever made up that rule didn't have a best friend.) Within seconds of taking my dear friend's hand and quietly speaking my name, I set off bells and whistles from the machines she was connected to that seemed to startle her even in her comatose state. Of course, I was asked to immediately leave.

My anticipatory grief was so severe I would not visit her again. I did not attend her weekday funeral as I had just started a new job and naively did not dare ask for a day off to pay tribute to my best friend. How stupid was my thinking! That is why I suggested earlier in this book that you wisely choose the funerals you attend. Thankfully, my husband Paul went to the funeral and offered our extreme sympathies.

After my dear friend's death and while severely grieving, I promised myself I would never have another close friend as I was not about to be heartbroken that brutally and abruptly again. True to my word, it would take years to change my mind.

Three years passed with me feeling sorry for my near friendless self. I am not sure why one day I decided that I needed and wanted to understand as much as I could about death, dying, and grieving. I became an avid reader about all three topics and found myself stocking my bookshelves with everything from near-death-experiences, to angels, miracles, and life after death. Soon thereafter I found the best nursing job I would ever have when I began working with hospice patients and families. I believe God had a very important hand in all of this, as my dear friend in spirit cheered me on.

A very significant part of my hospice life evolved as I began collecting and compiling stories told to me by my hospice patients and their loved ones, hospice staff and volunteers, neighbors, other health care providers, past acquaintances, and my own family members. Sharing one's story became a great way for all of them, and me, to find meaning and understanding of what we have experienced as one's death approached or already transpired. It has been also a great way for many to work through their grief by putting their story on paper…and having someone believe it.

Alas, I have finally reached a mature concept of death. My life is now filled with more friends than I have ever had! That does not mean I no longer grieve for my dear friend but rather I have accepted her death and have definitely grown as a result of it. I can not physically see her but I can spiritually feel her.

No Greater Love

The best of friends are undoubtedly those who are in a very loving and caring marriage, whether for five or fifty years. We could learn volumes from them about loving, living, and dying. Studies have shown that the death of a spouse may even hasten the death of the other; perhaps this is grief's greatest blow. The term *chronic adversity* relates to this phenomenon of when the distress related to care giving of the very ill has a negative effect on the care giver who may acquire or exacerbate diseases such as cancer, heart disease, diabetes mellitus, increased viral responses and even periodontal disease.

Startling results from research indicates that the caregivers of the terminally ill may in fact die at a notably greater rate that those who were not caregivers. Two very devoted couples come to mind: In 2004, Superman hero Christopher Reeves died at age fifty. He credited his wife Dana's love and her care giving as to what sustained him far longer than anyone predicted. Eighteen months after her husband passed, Dana died at a young age of forty-four. World famous singers/songwriters June Carter Cash and her husband Johnny Cash died four months apart in 2003. They were both in their early seventies.

In my own experience as a hospice nurse, *chronic adversity* played out in one of my young married couples. JP was twenty-seven-years-old when I cared for her. She was dying from cancer. She had a toddler son and a very loving and attentive husband. Just three months after her death, her husband died at twenty-nine-years of age of a different and rare type of cancer. He had no symptoms of the disease during his wife's illness or at her death.

Hospice nurse Linda Feiler shares her very similar story about her parents who loved deeply in life and death:

She was his 'Bessie.' Her name was Mary Elizabeth, but to him she would always be 'Bessie.' He knew from the first moment he saw her that she was 'the one.' That was fifty-six years ago. Fifty-six years of laughter, loving and living life together; fifty-six years of raising a daughter, caring for parents, grandchildren and family.

Bessie was the Matriarch of the family. The one everyone depended on for love, support and joy; chief cook and bottle washer, solver of all problems, and giver of so much to so many, especially to him.

But something had gone wrong. He had watched the light slowly fade from her eyes. Watched the person that he had known for so many years begin to change into someone without hope. Frantically, he searched for the cause and was told that she had Alzheimer's dementia. There was no cure.

That began a twelve-year descent into darkness for his Bessie and, the worse horror that he could imagine, the slow progression of the person that he loved more than life itself, toward death.

He tried everything he could- vitamins, medicine, exercise, puzzles. Every day, she had a routine that was consistent and so loving. He would wake her up by rubbing her back. Her first medication of the day was given and then he would help her dress. Next, he would try to get her to eat. Eating became more difficult with each passing day. Sometimes she would just shake her head and refuse. She became agitated and wouldn't sleep, wandering throughout the house, falling. Tirelessly, day by day, he worked to keep her going, to keep her alive. Finally, it became too much for even him to handle. He had struggled for so long and he was losing the battle. We were all there with him in the struggle, but it was his determination, his perseverance that had kept her going for so long.

He knew that he couldn't take care of her at home. He was worn out and at the end of his rope. That's when we called hospice and arranged for her to go to the Hospice House. It was so hard to tell her. She still knew who we were. Still talked to us and had moments that she knew what was happening. She couldn't understand why she had to go, but she agreed.

He couldn't do it. He couldn't take her. It was beyond his ability to cope. To take his 'Bessie' away was the hardest thing anyone could ask, and he just couldn't do it. And so, he asked me to take her, and I helped her to get ready.

I will never forget that day or how hard that drive was for both my mom and me. I had to reassure her so many times, and when we arrived, her anxiety continued to escalate in spite of the wonderful care she immediately received. It became apparent after only a short time that she would need much more care and she was transferred to the Hospice Care Center in Port Orange, Florida.

Mom was given the best care imaginable. It was so comforting to Dad and me to know that she was with such loving and caring staff. Dad came as often as he could to see her, but it was difficult for him to make the trip. He was so tired. It was as if he had used every ounce of strength caring for her.

Mom was in the Care Center two weeks. She always knew who we were and had a smile for each of us. There are so many special moments that we will never forget. So many good memories.

Dad's Bessie died on October 16, 2005. We celebrated her life in a wonderful memorial service with the help of hospice volunteers and family.

That was on Saturday. By the following Wednesday, Dad was in the Intensive Care Unit at Halifax Hospital. At first it appeared that it was a bad case of pneumonia. He was cheerful and celebrated his 80th birthday with many of his family at his side. He remained in the hospital for ten days, slowly losing ground, unable to breathe without substantial oxygen assistance.

Finally, we were told that there was nothing more to be done. He had a severe lung disease that would not improve. He could not live without twenty-four hour care and oxygen assistance. Even then it would only be a matter of time.

Dad said no more. No more hospital, no more oxygen. "I want to go to the Care Center. That's the last place I saw my Bessie." And so Dad was taken to the Care Center. When he arrived, he said, "Now I'm home." He died the next day, exactly three weeks after his Bessie, my Mom.

I write this for several reasons. First, to acknowledge a man who loved his wife more than life itself. A man who gave everything he had to love and care for her. He is my hero and always will be. Mom and Dad had a very special love and they were a blessing to everyone who knew them. They will always be in our hearts.

Mom's and Dad's story might have had a very different ending had it not been for the staff of Hospice of Volusia/Flagler. They provided a safe place for both Mom and Dad, and for me, their daughter. I knew from the first day that they would receive only the best of care, and because of the love and care I received, I was able to survive the loss of both Mom and Dad within such a short period of time.

I will never forget my parents. I will never forget those who cared for them.

John 15:13. Greater love has no one than this that he lay down his life for his friends.

Peaceful Angel

Another love story etched with compassion, joy, and grief is told by Mimi Pacifico, a hospice volunteer, who believes in and teaches about the power of end-of-life education and preparation:

Despite the fact that my husband, Angelo, was getting excellent care in the hospital, I was growing more frustrated every day.

His main medical problem was a heart not strong enough to do its job, affecting other organs, which I believed were shutting down. He had a specialist for every organ in his body and each one wanted to give him additional medication. "Why?" I wondered. I heard so many different opinions my head was spinning.

Out of town family members were frustrated over visiting hours in the Intensive Care Unit. One day, the nurse sheepishly appeared in the waiting room and announced Mr. Pacifico wanted to see all of his family at one time, NOW. That may have been his last assertive act.

Finding veins and drawing blood became an ever increasing difficulty. Chaos reigned. I knew it was time to call in hospice. The doctors were most supportive and cooperative. Within a few days, arrangements were made and Angelo was transferred to Majestic Oaks Continuing Care Community at John Knox Village in Orange City, Florida, under hospice care.

Without the struggle, he could say his good-byes, peacefully come to terms with and accept his final journey. Within a few days, with oxygen, pureed food and only comfort medications, he improved slightly. I knew it was merely the quality of life that would be different. Not the length of his days. Nothing could be done to strengthen his weak heart. The Majestic Oaks staff and the hospice team administered tender loving care, which he recognized and appreciated.

Some days my hopes were high. The next, they would plummet. His hospice team was there for me and for him, a constant comfort. He withdrew a bit more, even less interested in the world around him. However, I marveled watching him feed himself, actually seeming to enjoy his meals and snacks of ice cream upon request. But even eating tired him out.

Never losing his sense of humor, endearing himself to the staff who cared for him, he was alert, always wanting to know the day ot the week and time of day. He took delight when I brought our pet cat, Pumpkin, for a brief visit. He slept more. When he was awake there was a twinkle in his eye and some remark to indicate he was listening and could clarify a puzzle or answer a question.

The early morning nurses told me they often found him singing. Several friends came and sat with him, not engaging him in conversation or waking him, just letting him set the pace. Bob and Joan LaFleur provided a television for his enjoyment. Barbara Graham, an off-duty hospice volunteer, helped decorate his room with photos to create a homier, less sterile atmosphere. On one visit, Angelo asked her, "Where do I go next?"

"Where would you like to go? She asked.

He then closed his eyes, smiling mischievously, and began singing *Heaven, I'm in Heaven*.

He and another friend, Betty Stearn, discussed the return of his son, Phil, and a grandson, David, in a few days. "Yes," Angelo said. "They are coming for the requiem."

As I left him the night before he slipped away, he seemed so good I thought he might go on for quite a while. The following day, the one on which Phil and David were to leave, I left them alone to say good-bye. I told Phil I would visit after they were gone. When he relayed that message to his dad, the comment was "I might be asleep by then."

When the phone rang and I heard Phil's voice, I knew our beloved was gone from us to be with the Lord. "I'm coming to get you," Phil said.

"We were laughing, joking, watching a rerun of the Preakness Race from the previous weekend," Phil tod me. "He took a deep breath, let out a sigh and was gone."

I entered his room as two staff members gently prepared the body. Tears were running down their faces. Each in turn hugged me. He looked so peaceful, relatively healthy, his snowy white hair beautiful. He was still a handsome man. I gave thanks to God for his good, happy life and jolly sense of humor. Who but God could have orchestrated such a beautiful passing? In the arms of his loved ones, without pain, free at last. The three of us circled his bed and I offered a prayer of praise and thanks.

A sense of peace flooded through me. I am eternally grateful for the loving care by the staff, the hospice team and the many expressions of kindness extended to me. Our friends coulnd't seem to do enough to show their love for him. I had found "joy that comes in the morning" and experienced the peace that passes all understanding.

I was thankful for the last few weeks when my husband lived the meaning of his name: peaceful angel.

Golden Memories

Love stories get me every time and Paul Burrows has penned his into a beautiful poem for his wife who he so lovingly cared for prior to her death:

Why do I love you still?
I love you because we once built sandcastles together,
and then built our own castle with bricks of faith and
faithfulness on a firm foundation, blending into one life
both church and home.

I love you because we once held hands and walked the
paths of youth, and now in my golden, shimmering years,
your hand upholds me and serves me only and always in love.

I love you because we once dreamed dreams together and
doubled those dreams into 50 years of reality and reason
as we strived for peace in each life and in both, and we have
found that dream again just now in this gathering of friends
who have walked similar paths.

I love you still for each and all of these...but even more,
I love you still because you have always brought out the
best in me, and always given me your best... not out of duty,
but out of joy and perfect love.

I will always love you for your magical way of making a
moment seem like 50 years or 50 years as a moment.
To newly married persons, 50 years may seem like a long
time, but to those who reach it, it seems like a tick of the
clock in the eternity of a love filled life.

I love you still...today, tomorrow, in all the symmetry and
rhythm of this life and the next.

I love you even more, if that is possible, for your love that is shared with Jesus Christ who brought us together in marriage and leads us...alone or together...in the way that lies behind us and in the adventures just ahead. I love you because you love Him. We have become our own small Trinity with Father, Son, and Holy Spirit entwined in our marriage as if held together by beautiful golden threads.

For this I know, I will always know, I love you still.

Social Death

Most of us are able to make our own decisions about loving, living and dying. Yet dying may involve something more than our physical death. We may actually experience a social death initially, when one's mental state does not allow the usual everyday decision-making and participation in society, such as with Alzheimer's Disease. It may be very difficult to emotionally anticipate and timely prepare for a social and physical death as Robert Kamholtz portrays in his story, *Another Tough Day:*

It hurts and I don't know what to do. I'm looking right at her and she's yelling at me and calling me derogatory names.

"I'm doing what's right. Please try to understand," I plead, while trying to keep my anger and frustration under control. I feel my pressure going up and the pounding of my heart as its rhythm speeds up.

Her face shows confusion- then contorts in anger. With clenched fists, she screams, "No! You're wrong. You're an idiot. You're crazy. You're very sick. I'm calling a doctor.' She races to the phone, hovers over it but doesn't pick it up.

"You have to trust me," I beseech. "I know what to do."

"Are you God?"

"No! I'm not God- but I'm here for you. I know what you need."

"Are you a doctor?" she shrieks.

I try to reach out to her, to touch her but she backs away. "No, but I know what the doctor wants you to do. He verified that these are the pills you should take before retiring. Look!" I say, holding the doctor's scribbles in front of me and trying to get her attention.

"Here are his instructions. In writing," I emphasize. "Please read them."

She reaches out, violently grabs the paper from my hand and takes a few steps away from me. I watch as she stares at the paper. I judge, by the inquisitive expression and contortions on her face, that she doesn't understand what she's reading.

"Would you like me to read it to you?" I ask quietly.

"No! I can read."

"I know, but do you understand *what* you're reading?"

She doesn't respond. She keeps reading the note over and over again. She grimaces, walks up to me, crushes the paper with both hands, viciously throws it at my face, and says, "I want *another* doctor to…" She pauses for about a minute as a blank expression comes over her face and her eyes open wide. I start to say something, but I stop as I watch her nose wrinkle up and her lips distort and begin to move slowly, unnaturally. She stares at me and unintelligible sounds come forth.

I say nothing and wait. She appears to be in mental confusion and agony. I feel sad and disappointed that I'm unable to reach or help her.

Moments later, I sense that she is calm, so I produce another paper. "This is from a second doctor."

No response.

"Both of them said the same thing. Both are trying to help you."

I pick the crumpled paper up, flatten it out and read aloud the first doctor's instructions. "Take…before retiring." I hold two pills and a glass of water out toward her and say, "It's okay, please stay calm and take these pills." I place them on a table and step aside, giving her space. She bites her lip.

"The pills will make you feel better, and soon everything will be all right." I coax.

She looks at me warily, walks slowly to the table and looks down at the pills. "Are you sure these are the ones?"

"Yes! *They are* the right ones."

I begin to feel relieved and relaxed. I'm almost getting used to this scene. Although it has happened many times before, each time it seems to take a little longer.

From across the table I watch as she places the pills in her mouth, drinks the water and swallows them.

"You can get to bed now whenever you want." I assure her. No reaction.

I purse my lips and walk to her, but this time, she doesn't back away. I take her hand and gently pull her out of the kitchen. "I'll put the TV on in the bedroom so you can fall asleep watching a show."

"Okay," she replies quietly and we walk hand-in-hand toward the bedroom. Unexpectedly, she stops and we separate. She looks at me, smiles and wraps her arms around me. "I lo…love you."

A moment of pure joy overwhelms me and I grin. "I love you, too."

What hurts me the most as a caregiver is watching the steady decline in her comprehension and her ability to think and to say things like I love you. I feel frightened and worried, wondering if today will be the last time I will hear those special words.

Along the way to the bedroom, I close my eyes momentarily, look upward and say softly, "Thank You, Lord, for helping us to get through another tough day."

I am Dying

A holiday life review with much reminiscing provided Jeanette Surratt a way to begin her own grieving as her death approached. Her request to her hospice Social Worker, Renee Palmer, was to share her feelings with our readers:

I'm waiting! In my eighty-five years I have waited for many things- I have waited for nine months, three different times, for three babies but those times were happy expectations. I have waited in hospital rooms while waiting for good health to return. I have waited for teenagers to make their curfew home on time. I have waited my turn in the doctor's office with many options running through my mind but now, tonight, I'm waiting again but this time it's different- they tell me I'm dying!

The day I sat in the doctor's office I was in total denial when he said, "I think it's time for hospice." I thought I was fine, just getting older, and he was wrong.

I was angry and said, "Absolutely no!" then walked out of the office.

My daughter went back and made the arrangements but I still felt they had the wrong patient. Next came the wheelchair and the hospital bed! I have yet to sit in the wheelchair and it's been two weeks. Perhaps I'll get in it tomorrow.

The bed is a different story- I had an almost new double bed that I sold to a neighbor for $30 and threw in $60 worth of sheets! I cried that night as I crawled into that small hospital bed but I found out I could sleep better when I raised the head up. Yes, I could breathe better and they tell me it's necessary to be able to breathe. So even at times I am still in denial but I am breathing, at least for now.

There are times when I look out the window, I am on the 7th floor, and I have always said, "I'm over the trees and beneath the clouds". Now the trees are turning and some of the trees are losing their leaves. Will I be home when they come back? Christmas is forty-six days away. Will I be home for that?

It is morning now, had a good night, but as I wake up I lay there and start to think, *how many more nights?* The sun is shining outside the window, the trees are swaying in the breeze, the sky is blue with white clouds and my bit of the earth is very peaceful. As I get up and dress it all comes back. Are they right? Am I still in denial? Am I really looking at the end of my life? So many things now run through my mind. So many things I wanted to do and didn't get done. Life is really so short. Why did I waste so much of it? Then comes the guilt-why didn't I?

We seldom get a second chance. I always thought I'd do it later then later never came. Sometimes we'd take a ride, see something we'd like, and say, "We'll stop on the way back." Then we went back another way.

So now as I lay in bed looking out the window, I think of all the things I didn't do. And as I lived my life I thought I did a lot, now I know how many things I didn't do. So many regrets- people I didn't help and should have, people I should have fed and didn't, and nursing homes I should have visited as I always intended to read to people who couldn't see. Now it's too late. My life is almost over. The clouds, the sun, the rain… how much more will I see?

Thanksgiving will be here in two weeks, one more turkey. How I used to love that day with treats on the table, dishes of nuts around the living room, the smell of turkey roasting in the oven and often lots of company.

Then comes the big day, Christmas!!! Will I be here? Just one more tree and a wreath on the door, presents on the floor, and happiness abounds. As I said, will I be here??

How many Christmases ago did Don cut down our first Christmas tree? The war was on and ornaments were hard to come by but we thought our tree was beautiful. So many after that. The smell of the fresh trees and how they would shed, but then we went to the artificial trees. No more gorgeous outdoor smells but also no shedding. There were fifty-five years of Christmas trees together. Now two years of lonely, sad Christmas trees.

I know I should be grateful for all the wonderful memories- the smell of roses, the taste of sweet corn, the feel of a newborn baby's skin, the laughter of a child, the color of a rainbow, the smell of a new car, and the lotion on the man I loved next to me in bed. Memories? You bet. They will be with me as long as I'm here. So I'm grateful but I'm also waiting.

It's starting again. It happens every year at this time. The days are getting shorter. The leaves are falling, red and yellow, as neighbors are raking and burning them. And I get weepy.

There are sales now on turkeys and mincemeat pies, and everyone is planning Thanksgiving dinners. But no more is it my Thanksgiving.

I listen to menus but nowhere do I hear *rutabagas*. Don used to peel them for me and when they were ready he mashed them. He loaded them with butter- it was his specialty. They were so good. With Don gone things are not the same. I sit around and think of many, many Thanksgivings in the past.

So now comes the depression, and that will last till after Christmas. I miss the decorating for Christmas- the outdoor lights, then comes the stringing of the tree lights. Don would lay them out on the living room floor. He was so particular, everything had to be just right, and then the lights went on the tree. What a moment that was!

That was just the beginning. Such happy times then, now all I have are tears and heartache. The depression lasts until New Years. No more happy times but beautiful memories.

Hands of Hospice

Mourning the loss of a loved one does not conform to any calendar or predictable date line. The process of healing and coping after a loved one has died is uniquely our own.

What one may consider adequate time to mourn may not be for another, even if the loss is for the same loved one.

One of the great things that hospice provides is bereavement support on an individual basis and also in group sessions. Julie Eberhart Painter, a hospice volunteer, shares her experience:

Had I not become a volunteer with hospice and eventually helped in bereavement groups, I might never have had an important healing experience. This life-changing event is the shining light in my eighteen years of hospice service.

My parents adopted me when I was nine months old. My adoptive father died in 1968. He'd suffered numerous mini-strokes, heart attacks and setbacks that would have broken most men with his dignity. It must have been terrible to go from a healthy sixty-year-old to a frail shell of what he had been in only eight years. Yet, I don't really know because I wasn't there. My grandmother told me later about the day he died in October of 1968.

My father had been hospitalized with another heart attack. Every evening my mother stayed by his bedside until he was ready to sleep. She'd then return home to look after her mother, a healthy ninety-two-year-old (who lived to be 105). That last evening, when my mother didn't leave at the usual time, my father, always thinking of his wife and mother-in-law, said, "Shouldn't you go home and see to your mother?"

My mother had a strong feeling that she shouldn't leave. "I think I'll stay a little while longer," she said.

Within minutes, my father closed his eyes and slipped away.

My mother died in 1972, and I contacted my grandmother who had moved to Kearsley Homes, part of a complex at the site of Philadelphia's oldest building, Christ Church Hospital.

After all those years, she looked exactly the same. We had a wonderful reunion. That's when she told me about

Daddy's death and we resumed our grandmother-granddaughter friendship. She explained to the now adult me that my mother always thought she knew what was best for everyone and liked to run things. At that time, my grandmother's unconditional love for her only child, spilled over onto me. I was next in line. She gave me her 124-page memoir, which I read on the plane home. It and she helped me understand the family priority list. Based on the marriage vows, "...and forsaking all others cleave only unto him." First came one's spouse then one's children, then one's parents. It had worked for her and her daughter. But the traditionally dictate list hadn't been accepted for the third generation, mine, when I chose to follow my spouse and then my children, forsaking all others and cleaving only unto them.

My father and I had always been close before I left home. My greatest loss when we were estranged was not Daddy's physical absence, but the gnawing guilt that I carried with me. I had broken his heart. Instead of shifting into normal adult relationships together, we'd polarized. When my loyalties turned to my husband, he accepted it, but my mother did not. Because my mother didn't, her mother didn't. But that personal dynamic isn't what this is about. It's about my father's spiritual strength and incomparable aptitude for unconditional love. He crossed time and space with hospice's help.

In 1995, I had been a hospice volunteer in Central Florida for about six years and had become a co-facilitator in our bereavement groups. We were trying something experimental the day I had my revelation and special gift. I usually "catered the session," passing out information and taking notes and attendance so the facilitator could concentrate on the group. But this day I was invited to participate in something new that they were trying to help heal grief: Visual Imaging.

We were asked to empty our minds and listen to meditation music, then visualize one last encounter with the loved one we had lost, the one person with whom we had unfinished business.

My unresolved issue, almost forty years after my father's death, was forgiveness.

Daddy had been a forgiving man in his life, but our family schism was a big leap even for him. I'd seen him in 1957, and spoken with him in 1960 when we were moving from Pennsylvania to Texas. He'd just suffered his first heart attack and I wanted to speak with him before we left. It was not enough.

Now I had to conjure him on a different communication level. Generally my attempts at meditation result in my mind running a laundry list of "to dos." Real meditation had always eluded me. That bereavement group day in 1995, I agreed to try to clear my mind and "see" him with the help of our hospice exercise.

The energy in the room helped me focus my thoughts and I pictured Daddy in my mind's eye. It was a shock. He and my grandmother stood near the back of a vast room. His face was clear, looking as he had the last time I'd seen him. I felt that he could see me, too.

When the facilitator called time on the exercise, we were asked if we would like to share our experiences from our fifteen minutes of meditating and visual imaging. Many reported healing joy and a sense of peace. When I was asked what I'd felt, my answer was "an overwhelming sense of forgiveness." That was hospice's greatest gift to me.

A Child's Grief

Children go through a stage in their more dependent childhood when they don't like being alone so coping after a death may exaggerate their loneliness. So when a grieving child must temporarily leave their surviving parent it may cause a separation anxiety in a child that would not normally react that way.

When a child makes a significant change in their school grades or wishes not to attend school functions it may be a sign of grieving. This reaction is similar to a child of divorce whose parents were both there supporting him or her in everyday activities and then suddenly one was absent. The memories may be too strong to deal with in those initial days or weeks of grieving so absence may seem the best and most secure option. In an end-of-life class I attended, I also discovered the same distancing reaction in adults who had experienced a close friend's death.

Additional signs of grieving, whether in a child or adult, can include a diminished appetite, nausea, lack of sleep, depression, general body aches, restlessness and/or shortness of breath. If a child or adult already has an illness then their symptoms may be more extreme, such as with allergies.

Grieving Parents

Attending an unexpected death of a newborn infant is probably the hardest thing I have experienced as a nurse. The air is filled with a sense of shock and an extreme sorrow. A surprising statistic shows that the majority of stillbirths are near full term infants with the expectation that, even with an earlier than expected delivery, each was expected to survive.

If you are a grieving parent, I recommend you find a computer and research the site *Mothers in Sympathy and Support (MISS)* which is for parents grieving over the death of their stillborn baby or infant. You can also call *MISS at 1-888-455-MISS (6577)*. Along with a bi-monthly newsletter, *MISS* also offers camps for siblings, educational seminars, annual conferences, as well as a multitude of links noted on their web site that address a wide range of concerns parents and caregivers may have.

To begin some of the first steps in the grieving process, *MISS* suggests both parents be involved in their infant's funeral and/or memorial service, the burial decisions, and allow extra time to provide special closure. Allowing the family adequate time to hold the infant for as long as needed shows great compassion by the medical and funeral staff.

The importance of choosing a funeral home that is very sensitive to the special needs and requests of the parents is paramount. Grief counselors usually suggest that siblings be a very important part of the proceedings, perhaps allowing them to choose one of their own toys to be left in the casket, provide the siblings time to speak at the service if able, and to carry the casket if desired.

Keepsakes are crucial in bonding the infant with his or her family. The baby's identification bracelet may be a very important keepsake to remove before burial. Making a videotape and/or taking pictures would provide memories of a time span that allowed few visual keepsakes. In lieu of flowers, the parents may suggest that their loved ones bring a stuffed animal to the service so each can be later donated to a favorite charity.

Parents in mourning are not only faced with immense heartbreak but often financial hardships, as medical costs can be huge and long-term. In regard to stillbirths, the issuance of a *Certificate of Birth Resulting in Stillbirth* can provide an income tax deduction that could assist with financial needs.

Other concerns specific to stillbirths and infant deaths are the need for medical research to decrease the incidence of infant deaths and stillbirths, provide funding for educating those responding during the death crisis such as paramedics, nurses, and police officers, as well as the need for bereavement support for the parents, siblings, dear friends and extended family. Any hospice organization can also provide a great resource for bereavement support even if the infant or child was not receiving hospice care.

The Compassionate Friends is a nonprofit self-help organization that offers grief support for those who have experienced the death of a child. One thing that *The Compassionate Friends* sponsors in December of each year is the *Worldwide Candle Lighting* that honors the memory and the life of each child that has died. Their Internet address is http://www.compassionatefriends.com or you can phone 1-877-969-0010. Your local funeral home may also have a similar annual memorial service.

Disenfranchised grief

Expressing our feelings about our grief may be even more difficult if it is not accepted or substantiated by our society. If we don't talk about *it* then *it* didn't happen, right? Wrong!

The bereaved may not be acknowledged as one who should be grieving, for example, when a mother miscarries, has a stillborn child, or a family pet dies. Perhaps there may be a certain stigma that has already shunned the dying from our society, such as with one who has AIDS, has had an abortion, is mentally ill, is in a same-sex marriage or an extra-marital affair. The consequences of any of these occurring causes *disenfranchised grief* that can delay the grieving process if there is a lack of support from a compassionate community. Grief can be delayed even further if there is no funeral or memorial service to attend to and pay tribute to the one so loved.

Suicide- it is emotionally painful just to type it. I can't imagine the sorrow for the survivors who attempt to find meaning in a death of a loved one who has intentionally taken their own life. Anger, guilt, rejection, shock, denial, and shame are just a few of the many emotions that disenfranchised grievers can experience as they mourn and struggle with disclosing very intimate information.

The latest statistics reported in 2004 by *The American Association of Suicidology* lists suicide as the eleventh leading cause of death overall in the Untied States of America. It is the third leading cause of death for young people ages 15-24. The elderly have the highest rate of suicide at approximately 16%.

The American Association of Sociology estimates that for every suicide there are six survivors. Thus it is imperative we direct our concerns to a minister, teacher, counselor, etc. There is a vast amount of support and contact information available at http://www.suicidology.org/ or if you are in a crisis situation you can call 1-800-273-TALK (8255).

Traumatic Deaths

Deaths that occur suddenly and senselessly can cause intense symptoms of grief including a strong longing and searching for the deceased, shock and denial, survivor's guilt, a rage against the perpetrator(s), and/or a severe anxiety that may be related to a loss of security or fear. There is no doubt that the tragedy of September 11, 2001 comes to mind, as well as the wars our servicemen have fought, suffered and died in. Numerous school and college shootings, aviation disasters, earthquakes, tsunamis, floods, and fires are just a handful of recent tragedies that remind us of our vulnerabilities and our helplessness in preventing such catastrophes.

The unusual circumstances surrounding traumatic deaths may complicate one's ability to cope with their loss and find meaning in the tragedy. The overwhelmed survivor, who includes the first responders, may have delayed grieving, requiring a longer period of time to process the incomprehensibility of the tragedy and death that has occurred. With multiple deaths, bereavement overload may be experienced as the survivor attempts to grieve for so many at the same time. The elderly who have experienced the deaths of many family members and friends are also faced with bereavement overload, while anticipating their own death.

Any death can have a traumatic grief response as I discovered on a Sunday morning in my local hospital. While visiting one of my hospice patients, her daughter privately explained to me that after her father's death four months prior, her mother went into emotional shock, not recognizing her own daughter and granddaughter or recalling any memories their family had made. Because of a very high fever that occurred a day before my visit, her mother was brought to the hospital emergency room. Within hours, she began recalling all the events that had occurred prior to her husband's death and recognized her daughter and granddaughter who tearfully shared their story. What an honor to be witness to her recovery.

The U.S. Department of Health and Human Services has done a tremendous job in offering ways of coping and dealing with traumatic events. You can visit their website at http://www.hhs.gov/disasters/emergency/mentalhealth/index.ht ml or you can phone for assistance at 1-877-696-6775.

TAPS

A non-profit Veteran Service Organization called *Tragedy Assistance Program for Survivors* (TAPS) offers a great support system for the survivors of those who have served in the Armed Forces. Because these families must relocate immediately from their home of service, their support system of friends and military neighbors are left behind. TAPS can become a valuable asset through the use of their caseworkers, videos, magazines, grief camps and retreats, support groups, plus many other ways it provides hope and healing as families mourn. Their website address is http://www.taps.org/ or you can call them at 1-800-959-TAPS (8277) for more information and assistance.

The Empty Chair

When my best friend died, my love and friendship for her did not die but rather she became more precious on a different level. In order for me to continue on, I had to relocate her from my physical life into my spiritual life where I still maintain my bond with her. The empty chair at her family's table will forever be empty and it will be a constant reminder of their loss. Grief counselors suggest there is healing power in talking to that empty chair, or it may be to a headstone or a picture, as if your loved one is right there with you. It can be very cleansing whether you cry and/or get angry, or whatever your emotion, as that may be part of your so-called normal grieving which is uniquely yours.

A Farewell Letter

There is power in the written word and so letter writing may comfort those that mourn. Having the opportunity to say words that were too hard to say before and no time to say them, to ask for forgiveness, or to say goodbye can give you some closure that is intimately yours.

Joy in Grief

What sustains us in our sorrow is what sustained us in our life, and even in our anticipatory grief, the precious memories we have made, the joy in knowing and caring for someone so precious to us, so very much loved. So when you feel the burden of sorrow weighing you down then reach for those joyful memories and lift yourself back up. Find yourself a new friend or rekindle an old friendship and start building some more memories. Once you recognize there is hope behind the hurt you may find much joy within your sorrow.

6 Afterlife

Angel feathers, sense of angels, visions of Heaven, visits from loved ones who have passed, and an encounter with Jesus are just a few of the stories that assure me there is another life after our earthly death, known as *afterlife*. I believe, when our loved one's physical body dies their spirit remains. On a shrine in St. Augustine, Florida, these words convey this belief in transfiguration best, "...we do not see them, but they see us."

God's Dressing Room

The moment we die I imagine it to be similar to stepping into a store's dressing room, changing out of our worn out clothes and stepping into something that makes us feel so much better, newer. Upon our death though, it is God's Dressing Room we are stepping into where he can see us with all our frailties. As you pass through God's doorway you may be wearing a hospital gown or your own jammies, maybe your favorite jeans and t-shirt; it is possible you will be wearing your *original* birthday suit or a suit of many colors. Either way, it will not matter how you are clothed, what size you wear, or what the latest fashion is. Hopefully we have prepared wisely.

Stepping into the center of His dressing room, you have no fear because, like most of us, you have been taught for years what to expect, which is a sense of peace and love that is beyond our ability to fully understand. As you glance into God's 360-degree mirror, you are aware that He is gazing back at you, just you, as no one else can pass through the locked door you just entered.

Whatever the time frame you have been given in your earthly life, this is your moment to stand in God's presence and be released from your physical body. A beautiful similarity of this transfiguration from body to spirit is often compared to that of a butterfly being released from its cocoon.

Some folks have an assurance that they will enter into God's presence when they die. Others may question themselves as to whether they did enough, lived a proper life, or showed enough love for others to deserve a heavenly home. If we can honestly sing the century old hymn *It Is Well With My Soul* then perhaps our self-examination in our own 360-degree mirror can validate our entry into Heaven before God tells us it is so.

Jesus said, "Write this down."

There are many stories in the Bible about Jesus and what He taught, the words he used to comfort, and the questionable places he visited. Jesus also visits today, even though we may not recognize Him, as this true story attests to that fact! It was told to me by one of my hospice patients, Fred Legge (who is now in Heaven), and his wife, Virginia, while I was assessing Fred's needs on a beautiful sunny Sunday. Virginia wrote their story down for me to ensure accuracy in my telling:

On a Thursday morning, Virginia and her thirteen-year-old grandson were in the business office in the hospital working out the finances to pay for her husband's rapidly mounting medical bills. Her husband, Fred, lay in a hospital bed several floors above them after having his toe amputated that day due to his severe diabetes. Even sadder news was that Virginia and Fred had been told just days prior that he had lung cancer and his overall condition was very critical.

While Virginia was completing financial paperwork in the business office, a man walked up to Virginia and her grandson and asked her a simple one worded question.

"Illness?"

Thinking that was an easy enough question to answer and not that intrusive Virginia responded with "Yes."

Then he asked, "Husband?"

Again Virginia simply responded with "Yes."

The gentle man then asked his final question, "Cancer?"

"Yes", Virginia replied.

Then the man said to her, "Write this down."

With a skeptical look, yet honoring his request, Virginia did as he asked. He had her write down four scriptures from Revelations that she put on a sheet of paper (that she has in her Bible to this day).

He concluded with two very important statements, "That will tell you who I am. Your husband is healed from his cancer but his toe will not grow back."

Virginia was really in awe now, as she never spoke of her husband's toe being amputated. The man then left their side, not to be seen again.

Later that day she looked up the four verses in Revelations and each referred to the *Lamb of God*. Her husband, Fred, was discharged home the following Monday in good health. His recovery was deemed miraculous especially after repeat testing revealed that indeed he no longer had cancer.

Modern Day Angels

Hospitals seem to have lots of great stories within their walls that attest to heaven's existence. This story, told by a co-worker and hospice nurse Cheryl Maxwell, strengthens that belief:

While working at the local hospital on the 3-11 shift, I had the pleasure to take care of an elderly gentleman in his nineties. Mr. Brown was deeply religious and read his Bible frequently. I had been his nurse for several days but on this particular day he had received the results of all the cardiac tests he had undergone.

He stated, "Well, did you hear the news? They say my heart is shot and there's nothing more they can do for me." He then stated, "...but that's ok. I've lived a good, long life and I'm getting tired." I tried to give him as much encouragement and support as I could.

At 10:00pm, I was standing at my medication cart outside his room when out of the corner of my eye I saw two extremely tall, handsome men dressed in suits walk up to me. I was startled to see them because visiting hours were over at 8:00pm and all the doors except the Emergency Room door (where Security Guards sit) are locked. They asked very politely if Mr. Brown was in room 521. I told them yes, he was, and asked how they got upstairs without a security escort at this time of night. One of the men just smiled and said, "We just walked right in; no one tried to stop us." They said they were from a local church and had heard Mr. Brown was here and wanted to visit him. I asked Mr. Brown if he would accept visitors, which he said he would.

They walked to his bedside while I returned to my med cart outside his door. I heard them read scripture and pray with Mr. Brown. Approximately ten minutes later, they walked out of the room, said "Thank you," and started walking back down the long hallway from which they came. I turned my head for a second to sign off a medication and when I looked up they were gone. I thought to myself that they might have gone into another patient's room so I hurried down the hall checking the rooms. I went straight to the desk that sits directly in front of the elevator and stairs. The Charge Nurse and the secretary both reported seeing no visitors. Security was called and he also reported seeing no men of that description enter or leave the hospital that night.

I hurried down to Mr. Brown's room. He was still awake reading his Bible. I asked him if he had known the two men who had visited him. He said, "No, but I greatly appreciated their visit because they had given me such peace." I told him about the men literally vanishing and no one else in the hospital had seen them but him and myself. I told Mr. Brown, "I think we just saw two angels." Mr. Brown only smiled and said nothing.

Mr. Brown was discharged before I arrived the next day. I heard he passed away two weeks later at home.

God's Earthly Teachers

Throughout my lifetime, I have met many ministers, pastors, priests, and chaplains. Each has taught me much about God's blessings, living while dying, and the belief in a heavenly afterlife. The men and women of God I personally am grateful for and would like to acknowledge are Floyd Tyler, Elwyn Putney, Gary Fairchild (my brother), Bruce Aubrey (my brother-in-law), Bob Brown, Esther Robinson, Father Roe, Jim Smith, Donald Rose, BJ Bishop and the many hospice chaplains I have worked with. Through their teachings and along with the great authors I have read, I have discovered and believe that we all have the same Father God and He doesn't expect us to be perfect and none of us should claim to be. Some folks may not approve of how we worship or practice our religion or what our rituals are in honoring the deceased but those folks are not the ones who decide on our afterlife. It is our relationship with Him.

Finding our Way

I would like to share some very comforting words of Donald Rose, an author and pastor from the Bryn Athyn Cathedral, who offers a beautiful understanding of the afterlife:

People who are dying sometimes mention the hope of seeing their loved ones again. The Bible speaks several times of death as being "gathered to one's people." Genesis 25:8 If we go to those who went before us, how shall we find them? Some are confident that God will take care of that. Some wonder about it and need further assurance.

One method Jesus used to assure us of His care was to have us look at the world of nature. Look at the birds. Although they have neither storehouse nor bar, God feeds them. Shall He not much more feed you? And what of finding your loved ones? You have probably seen pictures of those seaside cliffs where birds by the tens of thousands seem to fill the landscape and sky. Although they are so many and although they may seem to look exactly the same, each one finds its "own." It makes its way to the nest, and meets its mate or baby chicks awaiting this miraculous return.

Emanuel Swedenborg points to the birds and animals being able to find their way and he calls this a demonstration that we can find our way in the world that awaits us. The marvels in visible creation can inspire us with confidence in the marvels of the kingdom of heaven.

Gone to Heaven

"We often forget that how a person lives, so a person shall die," says Elsie Hudome, a Hospice Clinical Director, as she begins her mother's story:

Mother, Mary Ellen Savidge, was always a strong individual both in body and spirit. When I was a child, I perceived her as strong, an authority figure, larger than life, believing even my Father would 'mind' her. She was physically strong as well. When my children were young she would hold one of each of their hands in her hand and then challenge them to get loose. They couldn't do it.

My Father died after a two year battle with cancer in 1966. My Mother was 51. She was furious to be left alone at such a young age. She had been abandoned emotionally by her parents as a child and now she was alone again. I lived a distance from her and even though we saw each other weekly, she felt truly alone. She felt like a 'fifth wheel' whenever she was around her friends.

Yet strength being her greatest strength, she started a new life and worked full time until she was 73 years old. She moved to Florida to be near me when our family began to drift to different states. She became a Hospice of Volusia/Flagler volunteer.

At 88, she had survived two strokes with minimal disability. Then she was diagnosed with lung cancer. She looked at me and said she wasn't having any kind of surgery or treatment and that was that! She would have Hospice of Volusia/Flagler when the time was right. My job was to decide when the time was right.

I began to notice subtle changes, eating less, taking naps, losing a little weight...Mother cautioned her hospice team, "things will be on my terms." And, "I like to kid around." For the chaplain, "you can visit but we don't need to talk about God." The nurse and social worker can "visit as long as it's lunchtime. We can have a sandwich together or watch some TV." The home health aide can visit and "wash a foot or hand or something. My daughter takes care of me and when she isn't here, my friend Karlene helps me."

Family from out of state began visiting at Easter. My son Mark, his wife Laura and boys, Mark, Jesse, and Connor surprised Mother with a visit. Around Thanksgiving time of 2005, Mother said, "I'm going to try to make it through the holidays." I have learned to listen well to people when they make such statements. It's like their soul communicates important messages. She had been doing remarkably well with no bothersome symptoms. My great fear was that she would begin to have respiratory distress. We had been lucky so far.

Mother loved Thanksgiving and Christmas food. Oh, yes, sweet potatoes, turkey, stuffing, all her favorites. Most of the family visited because we had those conversations about what Mother said about making it through the holidays. My son Chris, his wife Sandy, my daughters Colleen, Dianna and family, Jenny, and granddaughters Brianna and Melanie all enjoyed a great day. Mother ate everything and plenty of it. More food than she had eaten at one time in months. She sat at the head of the table and listened to all the conversations. She wasn't as talkative as she usually was. We were just glad she was with us.

Then came the crash. The day after Thanksgiving she did not fully wake up. She was in bed and not talking, eating or drinking for close to 48 hours. My son and his wife said goodbye and left for Washington State knowing this was the last time they would be seeing Mother.

Two days later Mother was up and eating again. I was very surprised, yet not surprised. Christmas was her favorite holiday and that was yet to come. She was always great at giving and what better holiday to give on than Christmas. My cousin, Richard, always said that she gave the best gifts of all the family members. I remember her saying, "Don't tell your Father how much this cost," after she purchased some wonderful gift that no one else would have given. My mother could juggle money.

On December 24th, Mother informed me that we needed to go shopping. She hadn't been out in the car in weeks. I offered to get whatever it was she needed thinking the trip would be too much for her. She said, "You don't understand. I can't send you out to buy your own Christmas present." We went shopping for earrings. When it came to a gift for me, she always wanted to spend too much and nothing had changed. I saw a pair of earrings with a small dangling heart inside a larger heart. The hearts were like my mother and I. First she was the big heart surrounding the little heart, me. Now we had reversed roles with me being the large heart surrounding her.

Ah, Christmas morning. It was the usual chaos, just the way she loved it. Jenny and Brianna were opening presents while Mother watched. She always opened her presents last because she didn't want to miss anything. The whole day was perfect and Mother was happy. Thinking back, she opened her presents without the relish she usually experienced. It was almost like she knew she would not be using her gifts.

On December 29th, after an unusually good day of eating three meals and a Wetzel's pretzel (huge pretzel from the mall), Mother announced she would be going to bed early. It was almost 10pm. As I was getting her ready for bed, she asked when Colleen and Brianna would be going back to North Carolina. I told her they would be leaving in the morning. She said, "Tell them I said goodbye. No tell EVERYONE I said goodbye." My ears perked up. That sounded like a message to me.

Mother laid down and shortly became a little restless. She kept her eyes closed but tried to sit up. I helped her up on the side of the bed. With her eyes closed still, she said, "Why hasn't it happened?" I asked her what she was talking about. She said, "Why haven't I gone to Heaven?" My mother was not a terrifically patient person, and I guess some things never change. I reassured her that when it was time, she would go. She laid back down. Her calico cat Sweetie lined her body up alongside Mother as she did every night and began to purr.

"Forty minutes later, my mother left for Heaven as my daughter Colleen and I held her hands. I was stunned at the simplicity of it all. No symptoms to annoy her. No long periods of not eating or drinking. Just lay down and check out.

Sweetie stayed alongside Mother until the funeral home came. Sweetie never really liked anyone but Mother. She ran and hid from everyone else and especially me because I took her to the dreaded vet for shots. After Mother was taken to the funeral home, Sweetie got into my lap and curled up. I cried onto her beautiful calico fur and she snuggled close.

For two weeks after Mother left for heaven, the sweet smell of her favorite powder permeated my bedroom. I don't have any of that powder in my house. Every night, when I go to bed, Sweetie lines herself up against my body and purrs. I wear my heart earrings every day.

This story is dedicated to Mary Ellen's family: Clayton, Elsie, & Jenny Hudome; Chris & Sandy O'Hagan; Mark, Laura, Mark Jr., Jesse, & Connor O'Hagan; Colleen & Brianna O'Hagan; Richard VanNoy; Patricia VanNoy; Beatrice VanNoy; Dianna and Melanie Heying

When Faith Met the Cross

While visiting Israel and Palestine in 2005, it was common to see signs and bumper stickers that said *Pray for the Peace of Jerusalem.* After reading Mimi Pacifico's story about her dear friend as she approached death, I better realized the significance of the prayer request:

In the dark of night, Margaretha Tenney's bedroom in Volusia/Flagler Hospice recently was illuminated with hundreds of medium-sized Christmas lights of green, red, yellow, and blue. They framed the ceiling and the arm of a metal trapeze extending over the hospital bed.

A ceramic Christmas tree stood on a small wooden table beside the bed. A Star of David outlined in brilliant lights lit up the wall at the foot of the bed.

Margaretha's family gathered to celebrate her 83rd birthday party. Twin daughters, a son, a daughter-in-law, a grandson and a granddaughter sang Christmas hymns and carols, blew out a candle on the birthday cake and opened beautifully wrapped gifts from their mother and grandmother. How much the guest of honor was able to take part in the festivities, no one will ever know.

During the night, a hospice nurse summoned the patient's daughters. "Come," she whispered.

"Mom opened her eyes, looked up, possibly seeing angels and was gone," one daughter said later. With her children at her side, Margaretha's passing was so easy, so simple, so peaceful.

Her early life was anything but. Born in the Netherlands, she worked with resistance forces during World War II to hide Jews, and to help downed Allied pilots and crew return to their units. In an earlier interview, she recalled riding across town smuggling concealed weapons to the Underground.

"I was 18 but looked 16," she said. "I was apprenticed to a pharmacist, so no one suspected a thing."

After the war, she married a Dutchman, gave birth to a son and twin daughters, and immigrated to America. Settling in Rochester, New York, where her husband died, she married a second time and eventually retired to Florida.

To her friends and family, she represented the true spirit of the Judeo-Christian heritage She knew what it meant for Christians to be grafted in to the ancient faith.

"Some people wondered if she were Jewish," someone said to her family, clustered around her that final day.

"Sometimes, she thought she was," responded her son.

"She really knew her Bible" was a comment often heard among those who knew her.

Margaretha lived what she believed. Her signature jewelry was gold hoop earrings, with a cross hanging from one hoop and a Star of David from the other. Her home was filled with mementos of a life well lived, faithfully expressing her beliefs. The bumper sticker on her lift van read *"Pray for the Peace of Jerusalem."*

Now in the cold light of day, the bed is empty. Lights are extinguished except for those on the Christmas tree. They burn as brightly as they did the night before, as though Margaretha's spirit still lingered in this silent room.

The Baseball Cap

Angels are known for their expertise when their believers prepare to pass on to Heaven. Reverend Joan Baliker shares her story about the work of angels:

Bruce entered a nursing home in 2001. During the move his favorite cap was lost. He was devastated since this cap was the one thing he had left that he truly valued, a remnant that identified him as someone special. Its logo patch identified him with the Chicago Police Force where his father had been an officer for thirty years. During his teen years he felt that he had assisted his father's work in small ways. After much searching through e-bay, another cap and logo patch were put together and he was happy again and wore it almost every day.

In 2006, when Bruce was moved into the Hospice Care Center, the cap was lost again. By this time he could hardly see, so when he asked for his cap, his sister found another one labeled New York Police and convinced him that it was his beloved, well-worn cap. He was satisfied and even wore it in bed where he was now confined with, among many other medical problems, a dislocated hip.

Fast forward now to Bruce's last two days on earth. He had lapsed into a comatose state and was not responding in any way. His sister commented that she felt his spirit had already left his body, but was hovering nearby. Still she sat at his bedside reading and talking to him. Joan, an interfaith minister and a believer in life after death, said to him, "Bruce, I know you are already in a better place and I don't need a sign, but it would be fun if you'd like to give me one!"

Then, getting ready to leave, she glanced outside the patio glass doors and there on a chair, surrounded by sun *light* and folded as only an ex-sailor would, was Bruce's famous baseball cap. Goose bumps covered her body, and she smiled. She knew her request had been answered instantly and all was indeed well. No one had been out there; the door was kept securely locked by his caretakers.

This sort of occurrence happens often down here at the Port Orange Hospice Care Center since there are hovering angels at work daily.

Priceless Memories

There is such comfort in knowing our loved ones who have crossed from this life to the next are enjoying the pleasures of Heaven. Ann Waris shares her story of such comfort:

When I was growing up, my paternal grandmother lived with us. She bore my father late in life and when I was born she was 93. Though she walked on crutches, she was an integral part of our family, helping my mother with the children and participating in family pastimes. She prepared vegetables from the garden for cooking, folded clothes, and performed many other simple chores. She arose at 4:00am. each day, made her bed and dusted before leaving her room. Every article in her room was kept neatly in its place.

She sang at family get-togethers, and appeared to have more fun than anybody else. The memory of her "clowning around" with the rest of us still causes me to smile. She was exceedingly healthy and remained active until a few weeks before her death at the age of 106.

I fondly recall the times she babysat with me while my mother helped with farm chores. Until the day she died, she never needed eyeglasses. She read to me from the Bible, Mother Goose Rhymes and Grimm's Fairy Tales. When she read, she followed the line of print with her finger, and my eyes followed along. By the time I was three I could recognize the words. I didn't know until I was older that running her finger under the words was her way of teaching me to read. She believed that most children could read at three and four years old.

One day when I was four, she sat in the yard, watching me play. I spotted a beautiful insect on the ground by her chair. It was black and when it raised its body to climb onto a small stone, I saw a brilliant red spot on its belly. Curious, I reached to pick it up. Suddenly, a crutch swung down and crushed the little insect.

I was both startled and heartbroken. She put her arms around me and stroked my hair. She apologized for scaring me and for having to hurt the "bug." Ever so gently she explained that it was a black widow spider and that I must never touch it. "It will frighten her," she said, "and she will bite you; the poisonous bite will make you very ill."

When we celebrated her 106th birthday, she said to my father, "This is the last time we'll do this." Momentarily not understanding, my father asked her why. Tears filled her eyes and, without a word, she turned and hobbled out of the room.

The next day, she called our family together. She explained that soon she would cross over to the other side. She said she didn't want us to be sad, but rather to celebrate the good times we had shared with her. Even though we were no longer children, she told my brothers and me to mind our manners and remember the things she had taught us. She reminded us to read our Bibles every day, so that we would "grow up right." She gave away her possessions, assigning gifts to each of us in turn. Her gift to me was a photograph of my grandfather in a wooly black beard and strange-looking clothing, enclosed in a velvet-lined case.

Grandma told us that an angel had visited her and showed her a vision of the Promised Land. She described it in detail: A rainbow of roses, zinnias, lilies, and orchids bordered the stately mansion in which she would live. On the grounds around the mansion were fountains of sparkling water and exotic trees. Angels stood on the bank of a crystal-clear stream, singing hymns and playing harps.

"The sky is so blue," she said. "It's hard to believe it. Everything is more beautiful than anything down here."

In the week before she died, she began to confuse reality with what we thought to be illusion. She would point and say, "See? Do you see it out there? Isn't it beautiful? That's where I'm going to live."

She died in July 1951, one month before my thirteenth birthday. She had been such an integral part of my life from the time I could first remember that, after her death, I felt as if a part of me were missing. One night shortly after, no longer on crutches, she appeared at my bedside and took my hand in hers. It may have been a dream, but it was so vivid, I'm not sure to this day if I was awake or asleep. She smiled and said to me, "You mustn't feel that I'm gone. I'm always near you, looking out for you, and seeing to it that you read your Bible and say your prayers." Then she disappeared.

A warm sensation washed over me and the loneliness went away. Each time I thought of her afterward, that feeling would come to me and take away my sadness. I'm 68 now, but I still miss her and when I think of her, the warmth still comes...and I still read my Bible...*almost* every day.

The Secret sent from Heaven

Many folks have told me stories about finding pennies or shiny dimes at a particular time or place, seeing a timely rainbow or numbers that hold special meaning for the departed.

The smell of one's favorite perfume or cologne or that special song may fill the air at an opportune time, reminding us of the spiritual presence of those who have passed before us. Pay close attention to the endearing reminders in your life. Kathy Hoffman and her mother had a special secret reminder:

I was fortunate to be able to sit at my mother's bedside and have lots of talks with her during her last weeks on earth. Her last month was spent in a hospital, very sick, with doctors telling me, "We have given her Morphine for the pain" and "We want to make her comfortable."

Comfortable to my mother was not dying in a hospital with an intravenous PICC line in her neck giving her liquid food. So off we went to Hospice House. I knew hospice helped people die but I didn't know they had a sixteen-room home in Fort Myers where people could come and die in peace. No tubes, no PICC lines, no IVs. Just beautiful rooms that look like something from the Ritz Carlton, good food was offered, and you could eat whenever you were hungry. Nurses brought their dogs and they wandered in and out of patients' rooms. The dogs always brought a smile to my mom's face and SHE DOESN'T EVEN LIKE DOGS.

Even at the hospital, watching television began to bother her eyes so we would talk. One day we were all alone. I said, "Mom, do you like roses, red roses? I mean, should we talk about this? If something happens, you know, like the doctors say, you might die, well, I would get you red roses, you know for the coffin. Do you feel funny talking about this? Maybe we shouldn't."

She smiled and said, "PINK," right away. "Let's talk, I want to talk. I love pink roses."

I told her I never knew that. "Well, if something happens, I'll know you would want pink roses. Since we are on the subject, Mom, you know I would bury you in your white dress, the one you wore for your Fiftieth Anniversary with Dad. I feel funny about this?"

"Don't," she said. "No, I want to be buried in my pink suit. I love that pink suit. I think I look pretty sharp in it."

I laughed out loud, probably a little from being nervous. "I am glad we talked, Mom. I would have picked red roses and your white dress! Now I know what you would like and that's what matters the most to me." I said, "Mom, well, could we have a secret, something just between us? I know it's going to sound crazy. But, if you die and when you get to Heaven if it's more than you ever dreamed it would be, if you're all right, and you see GOD, you see JESUS, see if you can send me one red rose."

It was a special moment between us, almost an eternal moment. We looked at each other's eyes and we both had tears. She smiled at me, only the loving smile a Mom gives, and said, "Yes, I'll do that."

A week later, I said, "Look, Mom, about our secret. I'll be on earth and you'll be in Heaven. How are you going to get a rose to me?"

She said, "Kathy, GOD CAN DO ANYTHING!"

Her mind started to go and so whenever we were all alone I'd ask her if she remembered our secret. She would say, "Yes, I'll send you a rose!"

I would say, "Remember what color?"

"Red," she would say, almost irritated with me for asking.

Well, once we got to Hospice House, I never reminded her again. She got sicker. It was such an emotional time. It had been one month since I had been home with my husband and family. It was tough watching her suffer and so I simply forgot about our secret. Now she wasn't talking any more, her eyes were closed. She wouldn't even hold my hand. The hospice nurses said the hearing is the last to go so I talked, I sang, I rubbed her face. I kissed her over and over and wept.

Finally, on September 16th she died at 3:25pm. Her funeral was in Ohio and she was buried next to my Dad. So many people came; they all loved her. Everyone told me what a wonderful lady she was and how she will be missed. She got over forty flower and plant arrangements.

All of a sudden in the back of the funeral home, I caught a glimpse of an elderly gentleman with a cane. I didn't know him. I was sure I had never seen him before. He had a sport jacket on and he had on a hat. I was in a conversation with someone when he walked by me, headed toward the coffin. I don't know why I turned and looked at him, maybe it was his cane. No, it wasn't his cane. What did he have in his left hand in that waxy green paper? I knew what it was in an instant. By now I stopped my conversation, I turned toward him as he knelt down at my mother's coffin and he placed in her hand just *one beautiful red rose.*

My hand went up to my mouth; in an instant I remembered our secret. I laughed, I cried, all at the same time. Then, I just cried...happy tears. She was in Heaven and she was all right. It was more than she ever dreamed it would be and she had seen GOD and our Blessed Savior Divine, Jesus.

By now everyone was looking at me; my two brothers came over to me to comfort me and to tell me to sit down that I had been through so much with her.

I told them they didn't know why I was crying, that they were happy tears. I said I had a secret with Mom. I shared our secret. I said, "Look, look in the coffin," and there it laid- *one red rose.* I'll never forget it. My mom and GOD working hand in hand to deliver me *one secret rose.*

I asked that gentleman, "What made you bring that rose?"

He said, "Oh, Honey, it's been on my mind all day; all day I've been thinking about it. I just knew I had to get one red rose for your mother."

I proudly carried that rose during the church services. After all it was for me!

A Hospice Patient's Prayer

Letter writing can be very healing for hospice patients and loved ones. Brian Murray writes this letter to his Lord while awaiting his passing into Heaven:

Dear Lord,

I thank you for the gift of another day. As I approach the end of my journey on earth, I am aware that each day is a gift from You. Help me to live this day fully, to be aware of Your Presence within me in those I meet today.

Give me the strength and courage to accept the challenges of this day. As my body weakens from age and disease, help me to accept these changes as a part of life and Your will for me. Give me the grace to turn to You as You turned toward Your Father at Your hour of need. I pray that Your will be done in my life and I place my body and my spirit in Your hands.

I thank you Lord for the many blessings you have given me. You have given me a long life filled with love and joy. I thank you for my family. I thank you for my companion and the life we have shared together. You have truly blessed me with all of them and I am very thankful.

I do not know when You will call me home to You Lord. The day and the hour are Yours to decide. I do pray for a peaceful death and I know and trust that You will be there with me. Until that time, help me to live my life to the fullest, being aware that this day is a precious gift from You. Amen.

Angels Among Us

Linda Farmer was so thankful to be given the chance to escort her mother part of the way to her heavenly home as death drew near. The people of hospice, who Linda calls the "angels among us", shared in their experience. After her mother's death, Linda wrote this very moving and comforting letter to her mom:

Dear Mom,

I know that you are in the presence of our Heavenly Father and sharing in the reunion with family and friends that have gone on before you. I am sure that you are worshipping at the feet of Jesus and that you are enjoying the light of the son on your face, while in the background the atmosphere is filled with the echo of angels singing *Holy, Holy*.

I have written many cards and letters to you over the years but I wanted to write one final letter thanking you for all you have done for me and for all you have taught me. Thank you, Mom, for the priceless inheritance you are leaving me, that inheritance being the knowledge of Christ. It does not hold a monetary value, nor do mere words describe its true worth. You not only told me who Christ is but you showed me by the example of your life.

You preached God's Word in a difficult era, an era in which women ministers were not accepted. That did not stop your determination to spread the Word; you went from tent meeting to churches and street meetings as an evangelist.

Your past was one of abusive relationships, loss, struggle and pain but you always kept the faith and always rejoiced in each new day God gave you. You are the strongest, most selfless person I have ever known or ever will know. You taught me to praise not only on the mountaintop, but to praise in the valley as well. You taught me to read God's Word and put His principles in action.

When I was a child, I would witness people treating you unkind at times but you were always gracious and responded with the heart of Christ. You were always generous and caring of others. You made sure anyone who visited our home was comfortable, well fed, and accepted no matter who they were or what their status was in life. I witnessed compassion and faith at its finest while watching you pray over an alcoholic father time after time, believing God would deliver him and loving him no matter how hard. I watched you give an alcoholic on the street something to eat and you would continuously put others needs ahead of your own. You found the best in people even when it seemed to be almost impossible to see on the exterior. You looked into their heart. You appreciated the simplicity in life and the simple things gave you pleasure, things others took for granted. I thank God that you are my mom and my example.

During your last days at home we shared so many experiences. I was able to serve you by being your caregiver and it was truly my honor. Thank you for the opportunity to give something back to you for all you have given me. I sang an old song to you that you used to ask me to sing when I was young. I was able to read God's Word to you for comfort at times when things were difficult and I was privileged to share your visions.

Although, I could not see the things you were seeing nor visit the places you were visiting, I came along with you in my mind. I would picture the places you were describing. We walked down country roads hand in hand. You greeted people that passed by that were familiar to you. We even sat in the cool of the day to have a cold drink and talk. That experience with you was very special and something I will hold in my heart and thoughts forever. You even asked that I draw a picture of my face so that you could take it with you. During the last week, you were able to see your dad and you described walking down a beautiful hallway and seeing the Heavenly Father's face with His brilliant light.

I have never witnessed the death process until now and, although it was painful, it was also peaceful and brought our journey together to a beautiful end. I was able to say 'so long for now' to you on an earthly level but also begin the anticipation of our reunion one day in the Heavens. Thank you for the memories Mom and for sharing your final moments on earth with me. I will always cherish our time together. You have given me so many things, not worldly possessions, but Heavenly treasures. I will miss you so much, no words can adequately describe my feelings of loss, but my loss is Heaven's gain. Your dedication will affect a thousand generations as God's Word tells us. You have planted the seed of righteousness and it will follow our family from generation to generation.

I will end this letter by saying, 'so long...my mom, my friend and my teacher.' You are and always will be the 'Wind Beneath my Wings.' I love you Mom. Until we meet again, your daughter, Linda."

Welcome Home

Countless times I have heard my hospice patients say, "I want to go home." It sometimes becomes a guessing game for loved ones to figure out which home is being requested. If the right questions are asked, it is soon discovered that my patients are referring to their Heavenly Home. I get such joy when I feel assured that Heaven is where these dear ones anticipate going and they will soon be stepping into God's dressing room.

With His approval, we will be reunited with those who have stepped through the door ahead of us. We do not have to be Mother Teresa's or Billy Grahams or a Pope from Rome to get into Heaven. We may have lived under a bridge with only the clothes on our back. Either way, the Heavenly Choir will be singing as Jesus welcomes us into his Heavenly Home. What an absolutely joyous afterlife that will be!

End-of-Life Caregiver Guidelines

E-O-L Publishing Corporation recognizes the need and desire you have to be prepared for your loved one's approaching death. To ease this time of transition and best prepare you as you care for your loved one, we have provided you with some signs and symptoms that may occur and some guidance in how to manage them. It is our hope that you have hospice care to assist you with any needs you may have. Please contact your doctor for medical assistance.

Anxious/restless- The one you are caring for may pull on their linens, toss and turn in bed, reach out into the air, and/or have poor quality of sleep. If he/she was an active smoker then a decrease in nicotine may cause restlessness. *How to help*: Play soothing music and maintain a quiet atmosphere, sit quietly, hold their hand if desired which provides comfort in knowing he/she is not alone; you may need to provide nicotine patches; make sure visitors do not speak inappropriately in one's presence as hearing is still present even if not acknowledged; provide a chaplain visit for spiritual needs if desired; provide a social worker if legal, personal or family issues are of a concern in providing closure; massage, aromatherapy or other complementary therapies may ease symptoms; the doctor may order a medicine to ease the restlessness especially if safety becomes a concern, if symptoms become more severe or to provide needed rest.

Breathing Changes- One's breathing may be irregular in rate and depth; apnea may occur which is the absence of breathing for 20 seconds or more; a gurgly sound may be heard in the back of the throat or breathing passageway; difficulty in breathing or shortness of breath may occur; loose dentures may obstruct ease of breathing. *How to help:* Reposition he/she to their side if able to tolerate it; elevate the head of their hospital bed as desired or use several pillows under their head; your doctor may order oxygen if feel it would be beneficial, a medicine may be ordered to dry up the secretions in the throat; keep your home cool to ease breathing and use a ceiling or portable fan; remove loose fitting dentures.

Confusion- The stated time, date, and place may not be correct; the one you are caring for may be unaware of those who are in attendance; words spoken may be mumbled or not clear in their meaning. *How to help:* Gently reorient the one you are caring for; speak to them softly while listening closely to their concerns/needs.

Decrease in oral intake/dehydration- As our body approaches death the desire for food or liquids naturally decreases; skin may become very dry; nausea and/or vomiting may occur; fluid may be retained in arms, legs or lungs if your loved one cannot process their usual amounts of foods or liquids; increase risk for aspiration (ingestion of food or liquid into the lungs instead of the stomach). *How to help:* Provide small bites of foods like popsicles, jello, pudding, or sips of liquids- cool temperature foods are tolerated better than warm; monitor for ease of swallowing; use moistened toothettes dipped in one's favorite drink or water to ease dryness of mouth- avoid using toothettes within the hour after administering medications that dissolve in the mouth; apply lotion to back, legs and arms if desired

Discoloration- Arms and legs may be pale and/or have a bluish hue; one's skin may feel cool; nail beds and lips may also have bluish hue. *How to help*: Provide a blanket, warmer clothing and/or socks if desired.

Fatigue- The one you are caring for may have increased drowsiness and sleep more with or without medications; he/she may not be strong enough to stand on their own or transfer to a chair- may only be able to tolerate staying in bed; may be in a semi-coma or comatose state with very minimal to no response to voice or touch. _How to help_: Let your presence be known with a soft voice and gentle touch; anticipate your loved one's needs that once were communicated to you; provide personal care that your loved one is no longer able to provide for themselves.

Fever- A high temperature or fever may occur; perspiration may be prominent during fever. _How to help_: Tylenol or Ibuprofen can be given; warm or tepid sponge baths are comforting and may lower the fever; linens and gown may need frequent changing.

Incontinence/loss of control over bowel or bladder- A decreased ability to release urine may occur causing discomfort and restlessness due to a full bladder; urine amount may decrease as the fluid intake decreases causing a darker urine color; bowel irregularity may occur as pain medicines often tend to be constipating and bowel activity decreases. _How to help_: Contact your nurse or doctor as a catheter may need to be inserted into their bladder; laxatives, suppositories or enemas may be needed; have a commode at the bedside if the one you are caring for is unable to walk to bathroom.

Pain- If pain control is a concern then medicines will need to be managed in the final days and hours by the caregiver; there may be more than one location of pain that needs to be addressed; pain may be exhibited through groaning, scowling or restlessness if unable to communicate verbally. _How to help_: Administer pain medicine regularly as administered before; if unable to swallow medicine your doctor can convert the medications to liquid or an alternative form of administration; remember you are giving medications your doctor ordered to provide comfort to promote quality of life at the end of life- medications are not intended to hasten one's death; call your nurse or doctor if any concerns or lack of pain control.

Visions vs. hallucinations- Visions of deceased loved ones, Heaven, or angels may be spoken of, the one you are caring for may reach out as trying to touch someone, talk about *going home* as they prepare for transition from this life to an afterlife; hallucinations with visions of bugs, dark places that are frightening, or other gloomy sensations may be related to a medication your loved one is taking and may be sensitive to. *How to help*: Listen carefully to what one envisions and don't discount it as false; ask who/what one sees and share non-judgmentally about it; if a medication is a concern consult your nurse or doctor.

What do the dying need most?

1. *To maintain relationships with those who are special in their lives and perhaps with those who have become estranged.*

2. *To know who will care for them in their last months, days or hours.*

3. *To listen carefully to their requests and maintain their dignity at all times.*

4. *To be honest and open with them.*

5. *To be touched.*

6. *To be allowed closure and time to say goodbye*

References:

Alfelt, Donnette R.,2004. *Comfort and Hope for Widows and Widowers*. Fountain Publishing, Rochester, MI.

Andersen, Margaret L. and Howard F. Taylor, 2004. *Sociology: Understanding a Diverse Society, Third Edition.* Wadsworth, a division of Thomson Learning, Inc., Belmmont, CA.

Balk, David and Carol Wogrin, Gordon Thornton, David Meagher, 2007. *Handbook of Thanatology*. Association of Death Education and Counseling, The Thanatology Association.

Boulay, Shirley Du, 2001, *Changing the Face of Death: The Story of Cicely Saunders,* Religious and Moral Education Press, Norwich, Norfolk

Brooke, Jill, 2001. *Don't Let Death Ruin Your Life*. DUTTON, member of Penguin Putnam Inc., NY, NY.

Corr, Charles A., Clyde M. Nabe, Donna M. Corr, 2003. *Death and Dying, Life and Living, Fourth Edition..* Wadsworth, a division of Thomson Learning, Inc. Belmont, CA.

DeSpelder, Lynne Ann and Albert Lee Strickland, 2005. *The Last Dance: Encountering Death and Dying, Seventh Edition.* McGraw-Hill, NY, NY.

Edward, John, 2001. *Crossing Over*. Jodere Group, Inc., San Diego, CA.

Harlam, Martha, 2004, *Dreamer: Diary of a Hospice.* Alicante, Spain.

James, John W. and Russell Friedman, 1998. *The Grief Recovery Handbook.* HaperCollins Publishers, Inc., NY, NY.

Johnson, Elizabeth A., 1995. *As Someone Dies*. Hay House, Inc., Carlsbad, CA.

Kirven, Robert H., 1997. *A Book About Dying*. Chrysalis Books, West Chester, PA.

Kubler-Ross, Elisabeth, 1975. *Death: The Final Stage*. Simon & Schuster, Inc., NY, NY.

Kubler-Ross, Elisabeth, 1969. *On Death and Dying*. Macmillian Publishing Company, NY, NY.

Kubler-Ross, 1982, *Working It Through*. Macmillan Publishing Company, NY, NY.

Lutzer, Erwin W., 1997. *One Minute After You Die*. Moody Pres, Chicago, IL.

Morgan, Earnest, 1994. *Dealing Creatively with Death*. .Zinn Communications, Bayside, NY.

Nuland, Sherwin B., 1994. *How We Die*, Alfred A. Knopf, Inc., NY, NY.

Saunders, Cicely, 1998, *Beyond The Horizon*, Darton, Longman and Todd Ltd, London, SW

Sykes, Nigel with Polly Edmonds and John Wiles, 2004. *Management of Advanced Disease,* Arnold Publishers, London, UK.

The FORUM, Association for Death Education and Counseling, Vol. 33, Issue 4, October 2007 Eldercare

U.S. Department of Housing and Urban Development
451 7th Street S.W., Washington, DC 20410
Telephone: (202) 708-1112   TTY: (202) 708-1455

Resources:

American Association of Retired Persons/AARP
1- 888-687-6677; http://www.aarp.org/families/grief_loss/

Association for Death Education and Counseling
http://www.adec.org/

Hospice Association of America (202) 546-4759
http://www.nahc.org/haa/

Hospice Directory- locate a hospice in the United States or
Canada at http://www.hospicedirectory.org/

Hospice Foundation of America
http://www.hospicefoundation.org/

Hospice Information- locate an overseas hospice
http://www.hospiceinformation.info/hospicesworldwide.asp

International Association of Hospice and Palliative Care
http://www.hospicecare.com/

National Prison Hospice Association
http://www.npha.org/

Parents of Murdered Children 1-888-818-POMC
http://www.pomc.com/

Survivors of Suicide
http://www.survivorsofsuicide.com/index.html

The National Hospice and Palliative Care Organization
http://www.nhpco.org/templates/1/homepage.cfm

About the Author

Judy Voss has been a Registered Nurse since 1973, is a *Certified Hospice and Palliative Care Nurse* and is *Certified in Thanatology*. She provides compassionate hospice care and end-of-life education to her patients and their loved ones, predominantly in Central Florida. Judy and her husband Paul reside in New Smyrna Beach, Florida.

Acknowledgement

It is with sincere appreciation that I extend thankfulness to the past and present Board of Directors for **E-O-L Publishing Corporation**: Linda Neider, Nikki Griffin, Doris Tomljenovich, Ann Bashista, Janet Ferreira, Kate Parker, Shirley Keesling, and Kate Ryan, plus deepest gratitude for Debbie Harley and Fran Davis of **Hospice of Volusia/Flagler**. Their encouragement and support have allowed the publication and worldwide distribution of three books that provide inspirational stories and end-of-life education, which have allowed countless patients a more peaceful emotional, spiritual and physical end to living.

Just as a butterfly joyously leaves its cocoon so too shall I leave my earthly body, my spirit soaring to places I can only imagine.   Judy Voss

Compassion & Joy